Bathing – the Body and Community Care

Community care lies at the intersection of day-to-day life and the public world of service provision. Using the lens of one particular activity – bathing – the book explores what happens when the public world of professionals and service provision enters the lives of older and disabled people. In doing so it addresses wider issues concerning the management of the body, the meaning of carework and the significance of body care in the ordering of daily life.

Help with bathing and washing involves nakedness, touch and the transgression of the normal boundaries of social life. Drawing on an empirical study of washing and bathing, Julia Twigg explores what receiving such help means from the perspectives of both recipients – older and disabled people – and careworkers, exploring the realities of work at the front line of care. The book deploys traditions of analysis from a number of fields, notably the body, but also historical, sociological and anthropological theorising in relation to diverse subjects such as time, space, food, gender and emotion, to present an account that radically challenges the ways in which we have traditionally understood community care.

Bathing – the Body and Community Care provides a clear and accessible overview of the literature on the body and its relationship to community care, providing an engaging text for students that will be of interest to a wide range of audiences, both social science and health science students, and nursing and allied professionals.

Julia Twigg is a Reader in Social Policy at the University of Kent at Canterbury.

Bathing – the Body and Community Care

Julia Twigg

London and New York

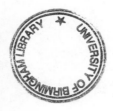

First published 2000
by Routledge
11 New Fetter Lane, London EC4P 4EE

Simultaneously published in the USA and Canada
by Routledge
29 West 35th Street, New York, NY 10001

Routledge is an imprint of the Taylor & Francis Group

© 2000 Julia Twigg

Typeset in Sabon by Taylor & Francis Books Ltd
Printed and bound in Great Britain by Clays Ltd, St. Ives PLC

All rights reserved. No part of this book may be reprinted or
reproduced or utilised in any form or by any electronic,
mechanical, or other means, now known or hereafter
invented, including photocopying and recording, or in any
information storage or retrieval system, without permission in
writing from the publishers.

British Library Cataloguing in Publication Data
A catalogue record for this book is available from the British
Library

Library of Congress Cataloging in Publication Data
Twigg, Julia.
Bathing – the body and community care / Julia Twigg.
Includes bibliographical references and index.
1. Community health care. 2. Community health services.
3. Bathing. 4. Body, Human. I. Title.
RA427 .T954   2000
362.1'2–dc21   00-042481

ISBN 0–415–20420–8 (hbk)
ISBN 0–415–20421–6 (pbk)

Contents

Preface

The aim of this book is an ambitious one, to change the ways in which we think and write about community care. Community care has been a neglected area intellectually, something of an academic backwater. Dominated by practical concerns, it is seen as essentially low-level and a bit dull. It has none of the life and death drama that attaches to medicine; and devoid of doctors, it has little social prestige. All too often its concerns seem mundane, lacking in intellectual challenge.

The intention of this book is to change that, and to set community care within a larger intellectual context. In particular, I aim to bring to bear on this territory, traditions of analysis that have developed in other fields, most notably those relating to the body, but also historical, sociological and anthropological theorising in relation to a diverse range of subjects such as food, time, space, architecture, work, gender, emotion, touch, nakedness. All of these have something to contribute to our understanding of community care, and deploying their insights will, I hope, help to widen the context within which the subject is analysed. Community care is about the ordinary and mundane, but this does not mean that its analysis should be ordinary or mundane.

Community care touches on some of the most intimate and important aspects of people's lives: their feelings about their bodies, their relationships with others, the meaning of home, the roots of identity, the struggle for status and regard, the fight to maintain independence. As such, it needs to be set in the context of a wider analysis of daily life and its meanings. What are the sources of these, and how do they relate to the patterns of service provision? Domestic life has its own rhythms and regularities, and we must explore these if we are to grasp the impact of community care on the lives of older and disabled people. How do they manage on a day-to-day basis?

What is life like once the front door has been closed and the professional – or researcher – has gone? Domiciliary care takes place in a special space, that of home. We need to grasp the meaning of this and, by consequence, the significance of careworkers coming into that space. Home is also structured in terms of time, and the patterns of this can clash with the logic of service provision, based as it is on a different form of time and a different, service-based, rationality. In the chapters that follow we will explore how these structures of time and space affect, and complicate, the nature of the care encounter from both sides.

Much of daily life turns around the maintenance and care of our bodies. Though we typically ignore such levels of existence in our analyses, our lives are in fact profoundly bodily based, and the rhythms of the body and its care provide an existential foundation for day-to-day existence. Grasping this fact is important in the analysis of community care, since it, above all forms of care, turns around the management of the body within domestic life. Though the management of the body is the central activity of domiciliary care, this fact has not been foregrounded in accounts of the sector, indeed, as we shall see, the subject has often been an evaded, even silenced one. The body remains a missing dimension in the analysis of community care.

This book in taking the subject of help with bathing and washing aims to explore a dimension of daily life that directly addresses these issues. Bathing and washing are practical, concrete activities, and they provide a focus for the exploration of questions concerning the management of the body at home. Community care lies at the intersection of day-to-day life and the public world of service provision. Using the lens of one particular activity – bathing – the book explores what happens when the public world of professionals and service provision enters the day-to-day lives of older and disabled people.

It is in the nature of care that it is created dynamically, at the front line. Bathing, like all personal care, involves close, intimate contact that can have a transgressive quality to it. How this contact is negotiated, the fine texture of the exchange is central to its meaning; and in the book, we will explore how recipients feel about receiving such help, as well as how the careworkers feel about giving it.

Though community care rests on the activity of careworkers, they have received relatively little research attention. In this book, we will explore the world of the front-line careworkers, looking at their activities as a form of waged labour. We will explore the employment situations that they find themselves in, and the impact of these on their day-to-day work practices. We will look at carework both as a form of bodywork and as emotional labour. Carework is often treated in a schizophrenic fashion, denigrated as a low-level job, yet also lauded as 'special' work, involving the supreme virtues of 'love' and 'care'. The roots of this tension lie in its gendered nature, for it is the fact that it is largely performed by women, and is indeed structured around expectations concerning gender and gendered identities, that lie at the root of its problematic character, and the diverse valuations that are put on it. In the book, we will explore the ways in which carework can be understood as gendered labour, and its parallels with other forms, such as nursing.

The book draws on an empirical study of help with washing and bathing provided for older and disabled people living at home, exploring this experience from the perspectives of both the recipients of help and the care providers. The study was based on interviews undertaken in two contrasting areas in Britain: a wealthy part of inner London and a decayed coastal resort and is described in greater detail in the Appendix. The study has been the basis of articles, and sections of the book draw on these earlier publications: 'The spatial ordering of care' published in *Sociology of Health and Illness*, 1998; 'Carework as a form of bodywork' in *Ageing and Society*, 2000; 'The medical social boundary and the location of personal care' in T. Warnes, L. Warren and T. Maltby (eds) (2000), *Care Services in Later Life*, London: Jessica Kingsley; and 'Social policy and the body' in G. Lewis, S.Gewirtz and J. Clarke (eds) *Rethinking Social Policy* (2000), London: Sage. I am grateful to the editors and publishers for permission to draw on this material.

I would like to thank the many people who have made this book possible. First and foremost, I am grateful to the respondents, older and disabled people, careworkers and managers, who so generously gave me their time. Without their willingness to share their experiences and views, the book could not have been written. I hope that it reflects these honestly, and that, although they may not themselves benefit directly from the study, its impact on policy and practice will improve provision for others. My thanks also go to Charlotte Salter who was involved in the early stages of the research. The study was funded by the Economic and Social Research Council, and I am grateful to that body and its anonymous referees for supporting the work. I also have intellectual debts. Though this is not in any sense a PSSRU style book, I have been greatly influenced by my time working in the unit at the University of Kent in the 1980s, and much of my grasp of community care comes from that period and the intellectual stimulus of contact, in particular, with Bleddyn Davies. I am also grateful for my time at the Social Policy Research Unit at the University of York, and in particular to Sally Baldwin and Gillian Parker. I learnt a great deal from working with them, and I am grateful to them for this. For me, this book is also a return to earlier themes, in particular to those concerning the significance of the day-to-day and the ordinary. My doctoral work on vegetarianism was undertaken under the supervision of David Martin, and I remain grateful for his enduring intellectual influence. Lastly, I have personal debts to friends who have read parts of the book, in particular Helen Charnley and Avner Offer. I am grateful for their stimulating comments. Above all my thanks go to Martin Peach for his unfailing encouragement and support, and his keen editorial eye.

1 The body in community care

Although community care deals with the most basic and everyday needs of people, the ways in which it has been presented often miss the concrete nature of this reality. Accounts of community care tend to be concerned with the institutional framework and the network of government polices that relate to this. These are important subjects, but the dominance of the approach has meant that much of the life has been squeezed out of the subject. The day-to-day reality of people's lives with its richness and variety is often missing.

This book aims to look at community care in a different way. These are three ways in which it does so. First, by focusing at the front line, it re-positions the analysis more directly at the point where care is actually produced. It is in the dynamics of the care encounter that the nature of what is produced is defined; production and consumption collapse into one another. Second, by looking at the practical activities of washing and bathing, the book reasserts the significance of the ordinary and the day-to-day. It is in the fine texture of these that our lives are located, and it is only through understanding such levels of activity that we can hope to gain insight into how services might impact upon them. Lastly, though community care is essentially about the care and management of the body, this fact has not traditionally been foregrounded in accounts of the sector; and the dominant approach remains a disembodied one. Exploring the provision of bathing and personal care enables us to put the missing body back in.

Refocusing at the front line

It is at the front line that the true nature of care reveals itself. It is there that it is created; and only there can it be judged. We can sense this truth through imaginative engagement. We can picture a continuum of care that at one end represents the best sort of care and at the other verges on abuse. Even if not involving positive cruelty, we can imagine rough handling, denigrating language, sneering or nasty words, a silent refusal to recognise the person, the demeaning exposure of the body, cold indifference to embarrassment or anxiety. At the other end, we can imagine the very best sort of care, where the careworker brings a sense of life and fun into the house, where the older or disabled person is encouraged and sustained, where what is particular about them is endorsed and valued, where care is structured around their preferences, and where lapses of the body are smoothed over. It is not difficult to imagine what these two regimes would mean for a recipient of care. To fall under one or other is to fall into two radically different worlds. And yet both can be described from the outside in similar terms. In both cases, certain tasks are accomplished, an hour of home care received. It is in the fine texture of the exchange that the essence lies. How care is delivered, how the service is forged at the front line is of central significance. And yet we know remarkably little about this front line. Domiciliary care in large measure still takes place in a black box.

This lack of knowledge has implications for the planning and delivery of community care. Currently the institutions of community care operate on an assumption that 'care' is unproblematic. In managerial and policy documents, it is often presented in terms of units of service, hours of the workers' time; and there is an implicit assumption that if you recruit the right person, all will be well and a standard amount of 'care', whatever that is, will be delivered. But the nature of care is more complex that this account would suggest. Care is not something that is produced back at headquarters; rather it is created dynamically, at the front line. As with other forms of service work, the processes of production and consumption collapse into one another. Care is not just given; it is also received; and indeed the very processes that create 'care' are interactive, dynamic ones. In order to understand the character of these processes we need to look at them from both sides, from the perspectives of both the recipients and givers of care. Care is thus not a simple 'thing'.

If the front line of care is so significant, why has it not occupied the centre stage of analysis? The site where it occurs is crucial in explaining this. Community care takes place in a special space, that of home and this, and the norm of privacy that applies there, puts limits on our knowledge. At the simplest level it is hard to gain entry into people's domestic space. It can only be achieved with their agreement, and even then the nature of the social encounter restricts the methodology, effectively limiting it to interviews. Ethnographic and observational studies of older people in their own homes scarcely exist. Such studies as there are are largely confined to institutional settings where access can be negotiated officially and where the presence of the researcher is sanctioned by the semi-public nature of the space.

Research has all too often reflected the values of the service world. Much of the work on community care has focused on the views of higher status actors like policy makers, care managers, social work professionals. The nearer you get to the front line and the lowly-trained, poorly-paid workers who actually deliver the care, the weaker the evidence gets. Research has also been biased by the scope and intensity of the service gaze. The more service dominated an area is, the more we know about it, and the more we attend to it in research terms. From the viewpoint of the policy world, it is service provision rather than day-to-day life that matters. As a result we know most about institutionally-based services and those where professionals are numerous and dominate. We know least about those services that are far from the gaze of the service provider, obscured in the private world of home.

Home care and the provision of bathing provide classic examples of these biases. Despite the fact that home care represents the largest part of the non-institutional budget of social services, it has received relatively little policy or research attention. The literature on home care is sparse, and little of it addresses the concrete nature of the activity. Personal care has been similarly neglected as a subject, despite the fact that it lies at the heart of complex packages of care and is a crucial element in enabling older and disabled people to remain living at home – the key policy objective of the last three decades. Personal care has partly been neglected because policy analysts have been squeamish in pursuing these private, bodily areas; and in the chapters that follow, I will try to get behind the screens of policy decorum to explore more fully the nature of personal care.

Re-valuing the mundane

As Siegfried Giedion wrote in his classic account of the impact of mechanisation on daily life which includes a section on bathing: 'for the historian, there are no banal things' (Giedion 1948, p. 3). The same is true for the social scientist, and one of the purposes of this book is to reassert the significance of the day-to-day and the mundane. Such levels of analysis have traditionally been neglected in accounts of community care. We need to explore them, however, if we are to grasp something of the day-to-day textures of people's lives and the sources of implicit meaning and significance that are embedded in them. Activities like bathing and washing play a central part in domestic life. They are one of a number of forms of body maintenance that permeate our lives. The round of getting up, dressing, eating, sleeping, excreting provides the bedrock of social existence, the fundamental structures that order our day-to-day existence. These activities, however, exist at a level that is rarely brought into conscious articulation or review; indeed in modern western societies we are largely educated to ignore them, regarding them as too trivial or too private for comment. But such activities offer a rich source of implicit meaning in people's lives, sustaining and expressing relationships, endorsing values and beliefs, providing an existential coherence to individuals' lives.

We can see this clearly in relation to the parallel area of food and food practices. Until the 1980s food was a neglected topic within sociology, considered too mundane, too much a matter of common sense, to be of interest to a discipline concerned with higher-status sources of power and meaning. The shift towards a new interest in the household and the private sphere, largely engineered by feminism, however opened up possibilities for exploring the significance of everyday life; and the new focus on food formed part of this (Murcott 1983, Twigg 1983, Charles and Kerr 1988, Wood 1995, Lupton 1996, Beardsworth and Keil 1997, Bell and Valentine 1997). As a result we can now see how food and food practices underwrite social structures, reinforcing relations of power and authority within the family and more widely. Diets and dieting offer regimens of health and well being that bring a daily coherence to people's lives. Through ideologies such as vegetarianism, food and food avoidances can be linked to wider political, philosophical, and spiritual ideas, embodying and reinforcing these values on a day-to-day basis. Food thus plays a central part in existential order.

Bathing and washing present a parallel, though perhaps less obvious, example of such meanings embedded in the day-to-day; and in Chapter 2, I will explore the history of these activities in the west and their links to the development of modernity. Part of the purpose of this chapter is to destabilise our common-sense understanding of what bathing and washing are about. Bathing has historically been located in a variety of discourses, of which the discourse of hygiene is not the sole or even always the dominant one. Bathing has had many meanings. Exploring these historically enables us to gain access to aspects of current practice that might otherwise remain hidden. For example, baths have often been used as rites of passage into institutions; and something of this sense remains in relation to their use by individuals at home to mark the passage of the day or week. Baths also have a history as part of coercive techniques designed to produce docile bodies; and being given a bath at home or in an institution can contain this sense, in potentiality at least. Historical trends in the treatment of the body also reflect wider shifts within society associated with High Modernity, and I will explore how these have consequences for the management of the body in disability.

By focusing on a specific activity like bathing we can also gain some access to the day-to-day lives of older people. How do they manage, how do they structure their days, what part does body care play in this? Looking at bathing enables us to see something of how domestic life works. The domestic ordering of life has a profound significance for our sense of self and of being in the world. In Chapter 4, we will explore the spatial and temporal ordering of the home, and the consequences for these of the coming of care.

The body in community care

Though there has been an explosion of work on the body in the last decade, this has not been reflected in the literature on community care. There are a number of reasons for this. One concerns ways in which the subject has traditionally been described and analysed. The dominant discourses constructing the field have been those of social work and managerialism. Social work has however never wholly claimed community care (as it has work with children and families) and its emphasis on casework and interpersonal relationships means that its theorising traditionally stops short of the body. Furthermore since the 1980s and the rise of the New Public Management (Ferlie *et al.* 1996), community care has increasingly been dominated by a managerialist discourse that stresses issues of efficiency and effectiveness, and focuses, in relation to home care, on allocation and targeting, and in which the day-to-day realities of low level carework are overlooked. Managerialist discourse is itself notably disembodied, drawing on traditions like economics, accountancy and organisation and methods that prize abstraction and emotional distance. The body has little place in these analyses; indeed it represents just those qualities of embedded, messy, concreteness that such forms of analysis aim to transcend. Managerial accounts of home care are notable for their disembodied, aetherialising quality;

and it is hard from reading them to gain any real sense of what the work entails.

A second reason for the neglect of the body as a topic in community care arises from the concern of social gerontology to avoid the excessive focus on the body and its decline that is characteristic of the biomedical model that dominates both professional and popular accounts of aging. In this, older people are defined in terms of their bodies and their malfunctioning. Much of the success of the Political Economy Approach within gerontology in the last twenty years has derived from its capacity to transcend this bodily emphasis and locate the problems of older people, not in their declining physical capacities, but in the surrounding social and economic structures that result in them being differentially poor, marginalised, and lacking in social and material resources (Townsend 1986, Phillipson and Walker 1986, Minkler and Estes 1991). The desire to avoid an oppressive identification of older people with the body and its decline is compounded by what Andrews (1999) terms the seductiveness of agelessness: the model of aging that denies the significance of the body and emphasizes the eternally young self below the mask of age. This has been influential in both popular and academic accounts that have sought to present a positive account of aging. Some theorists have argued for a radically social constructionist approach to old age that denies the relevance of the physical body altogether.

Similar processes have occurred within the disability movement where since the 1980s there has been a conscious attempt to get away from an emphasis on the bodies of disabled people – their failure, their dysfunctionality – and seek instead the social sources of disability. An emphasis on the bodily is seen as potentially demeaning to disabled people. At worst it presents them as the rejected Other of the freak show, subject to the prurient, pitying gaze of dominant society; and disabled women in particular have written of the distress and anger caused by being the subject of a voyeuristic speculation on what is 'wrong' with their bodies (Morris 1993, Lonsdale 1990). The Social Model of Disability, associated with the work of Oliver, Finkelstein and others, offered a way of getting away from this narrow focus on impairment, asserting instead that it was society not the body that disabled people (Oliver 1990, Morris 1993). More recently, this dominant framework has itself been subject to critique. Hughes and Paterson (1997) argue that the social model by looking only at disability, consigned the bodily (in the form of impairment) to the theoretical shadows, or worse the realm of bio-medicine, leaving large parts of the subjective experience of disabled people invisible and untheorised. Work by Shakespeare (1994), Hughes and Paterson (1997) and others has begun to explore the possibilities of using post-structuralist and phenomenological approaches to the body to develop a sociology of impairment.

Just as social gerontology and disability studies have been slow to take up the issue of the body so too the new sociology of the body, which has exploded over the last decade, has been reluctant to apply its analyses to older people. With the exception of pioneering work by Featherstone and Hepworth (1991) (and latterly Öberg (1996) and Katz (1996)) writing about the body has emphasised younger, sexier bodies. In part this reflects the way the subject emerged out of feminist and queer theorising around the construction of sexualities and the status of the body in this, but the bias towards youth also reflects a more general bias in the representation and treatment of bodies in culture: it is not just in academic literature that older bodies are absent.

The mainstream literature on the body is also marked by the remnants of an older cultural conflict in which the body's worth and goodness is asserted against what is perceived as an enduring Manichean strain in western culture. This discourse of the 'good body' is part of a wider twentieth century secularising project in which bodily pleasure, desire and freedom are asserted against what is presented as a repressive past; and it has links with the postmodern presentation with the body as a site of consumption and pleasure (Featherstone 1991). This consciously up-beat, positive emphasis, however, is ill-at-ease when faced with what I will term 'the negativities of the body' – dirt, decay, decline, death – and it is precisely these negativities that lie at the core of some at least of the experience of aging, however much positive accounts may wish to downplay them.

The desire to emphasise the positive and to downplay the darker side of care is a established part of the progressivism of social policy as a discipline. Emphasising models of good practice, focusing on user empowerment, promoting normalisation, eradicating oppressive language: all have been part of attempts by reformist bodies and individuals to improve practice through presenting it within an optimist framework. (The work of the Joseph Rowntree Foundation with its active promotion of such frameworks through its research agenda is an example of this.) But such consciously upbeat ap-proaches frequently involve presenting an idealised account that suppresses the darker realities of care. Smith and Brown (1992) argue that such processes of self censorship have been central to movements like normalisation where images and language are controlled in pursuit of a more positive approach, and that this has led the social policy literature to deny the darker elements in carework.

In the chapters that follow we will explore the ways in which bodily themes resonate through the subject of community care. Before doing so, however, we need to review the main elements of the new literature on the body.

New interest in the body

The new interest in the body that has sprung up across the arts and social sciences in the last decade has its roots in a complex set of intellectual and social influences. All start in some degree, however, from a dissatisfaction with the dominant rationalistic account that has characterised the social sciences since their inception in the eighteenth century. Social science is part of the Enlightenment project that has privileged the rational, controlled and abstract over the disordered, uncontrolled and concrete. In this intellectual process, emotions and the body were relegated to a secondary status and a discredited (and as we shall see, gendered) set of categories. Sociology in particular, in its struggle to establish its own intellectual territory and to throw off the spectre of biological reductionism, engaged as a distancing exercise, in which the conceptual realm of the *social* was secured and established by means of excluding the *biological* and handing that over to science. The price of this exercise of disciplinary definition was however, Turner argues in his ground-breaking book of 1984, the effective exclusion of the body and its concerns from sociological analysis (Turner 1984, 1991, Williams and Bendelow 1998). The body came to be seen as distinct from the rational actor, something to be transcended or ignored. The legacy of the rational actor has been particularly strong in certain social sciences, notably economics and in its related practical fields such as management sciences. In so far as topics like social services have fallen under the influence of such thinking, this has acted as a break on the development within them of theorising on the body.

Not all sociological theorising in the past excluded the body, and Turner has outlined an oppositional tradition from Nietzsche through Schopenhauer to Marcuse and Foucault in which the body, as the seat of desire, irrationality and pleasure, offers the basis for a radical critique of capitalist rationality (Turner 1991). The pedigree is a complex one and encompasses a range of contradictory theorists.

All however are united in their critique of the narrow rationality of the dominant social science paradigm.

The most sustained challenge to the rationalistic account has come from feminism. From its inception, feminism has been concerned to show the ways in which women's bodies are controlled and manipulated within patriarchy, focusing on a range of issues from abortion and reproductive rights, through rape, pornography and the wider media commodification of women's bodies, to dieting and the imposition of beauty ideals (Martin 1987, Smart 1989, Wolf 1990, Lovenduski and Randall 1993, Davis 1995, 1997). A series of social institutions – medicine, religion, marriage, the law – are implicated in the control of women, through the control of their bodies. Patriarchy was shown to operate directly on and through the bodies of women (Walby 1990). This was not just a matter of representation, but extends to the physicality of the body itself. Women, as Young (1990) showed in her seminal essay 'Throwing like a Girl', are encouraged to develop bodies that are weak, hesitant, reactive and soft; and this is in contrast to the active bodily confidence encouraged in men. These gendered differences, particularly around diffidence and modesty, have consequences for the experience of the body in relation to care.

Feminism has also been concerned to explore the ways in which women have been presented within culture as more embodied than men – to the extent that they come to represent the Body itself – and the ways in which this has been used to justify exclusionary practices (Jordanova 1989, Bashford 2000). Women are reduced to their bodies, confined within the matrixes of sexuality and reproduction. Women's bodies have traditionally been presented negatively as lesser, in some sense pathological compared with the male norm: fluid, soft, weak, uncontrolled and leaky compared with the hard, strong defined, contained bodies of men. Women are caught in a set of dichotomies in which they represent the devalued, unmarked, silenced categories of nature, the body, the emotions in contrast to culture, the mind, reason.

Malestream sociology has by and large reflected and endorsed this negative account, and this has had consequences for the analysis of areas of life in which the body and the emotions are to the fore. Davies (1995), for example, notes how traditional Weberian rationality is ill-adjusted to deal with the nature of nursing work. Waerness (1987) has made a similar point in relation to care, attempting to develop a rival rationality – a rationality of caring. The feminist project has aimed to bring the body and emotion back in, and in ways in which its truths and experiences are valued not repressed. Feminism has sought a fuller more satisfactory account of being than the over-rational, controlled and limited one presented in the dominant analytic tradition. In doing so it has opened up possibilities of exploring men's experiences of embodiment too (Connell 1995). Focusing on issues of violence, aggression, war, sexuality (especially gay sexuality) this new gendered perception has, however, been slow to move as Morgan (1993) advocated beyond a narrow 'over-phallusised picture of man' to encompass the bodies of not just athletes and soldiers but dons and bishops also. This is important for the development of a sociology of embodiment in old age, since the earlier emphasis on strength, violence and virility is not particularly helpful in the analysis of the bodily experiences of older men. Feminist accounts of the body have similarly avoided the experiences of older women, though new work by Furman and others has begun to redress this (Furman 1997, Ginn and Arber 1993, Featherstone and Wernick 1995).

The interest in embodiment has encouraged a parallel interest in emotion (James and Gabe 1996, Bendelow and Williams 1998). Emotion occupies an uncertain position within the sociology of the body. Some feelings – desire, anger – seem to belong relatively naturally in this territory; others – amusement, boredom – less obviously so. The reason for this uncertainty is that emotions lie at the crux of the central intellectual problem of the area, that of the mind/body divide. As many commentators remark, we both *are* and *have* our bodies. Hyphenated terms such as bio-social, psycho-somatic and psycho-social represent attempts to express this co-existence of mind, body and society, but at the same time they testify to the 'radical disconnectedness of our thoughts' (Kontos 1999). Literature about the body and embodiment has struggled with the legacy of Cartesian dualism. Although various attempts have been made to transcend these dichotomies, none has proved wholly stable or satisfactory, and the issue remains to haunt the sociology of the body (Williams and Bendelow 1998).

Recent sociological work on emotions has tended to avoid these kinds of theoretical issues and concentrates on the deployment of emotion in social life, particularly in work. Hochschild's account of flight attendants was a seminal study here, and her characterisation of emotional labour has been extended in fields such as hospice work, nursing and carework generally (Hochschild 1983, James 1989, 1992, Lee-Treweek 1996). Here the issues are less those of the body itself than the role of emotion in social life, though it is important to note that many of the areas where emotional labour is of central significance are also ones where bodywork and body care are involved. Once again gender is the key. Definitions of 'women's work', both paid and unpaid, are often rooted in ideas of women's essential nature as more emotional, more bodily, so that the link between body work and emotion is directly maintained in the person of the woman worker. We will explore these links in Chapters 7 and 8 when we discuss the nature of carework as bodywork and as emotional labour.

Perhaps the most significant single influence on work on the body has been that of Foucault (1973, 1977, 1979). For Foucault, history is the history of bodies. The body is the ultimate site of the exercise of political and ideological control; and it is the surveillance, regulation and disciplining of bodies, thereby rendering them docile, useful and productive that lies at the heart of his vision of society. For Foucault, the body itself has no pre-discursive existence; there is no natural body underlying social processes, rather it is created through the processes of discourse themselves. It is thus historically contingent and can only be studied by means of the history of the discourses that have formed it (Sheridan 1980, Rabinow 1984, Merquior 1985, Williams and Bendelow 1998).

Foremost among these have been those relating to medicine. The emergence of the teaching hospital – Foucault's Birth of the Clinic – played a pivotal point in the conceptualisation of the body in the West. The rise of a systematic anatomy, the development of physical examination, the invention of new means of observing and monitoring the body such as the stethoscope and the X-ray, allowed the body to be known in new ways. For Foucault the medical encounter is the supreme example of surveillance in which the body becomes an object to be viewed, touched, explored, penetrated and laid open, made subject to the medical gaze. These developments were not confined to the hospital but occurred across a range of social institutions and systems of knowledge: the prison, the school, the poor house, the factory. Bentham's panopticon provides the paradigm of these disciplinary processes whereby individuals in the prison are made subject to detailed and continuous surveillance from a disembodied and all seeing eye at the heart of the institution. In prison the body and its intimate needs for food, light, space, privacy, sex become the material on which the regime of schedules, curfews, denials, micropunishments are enacted. Thus from the organisation of architectural space, through the temporal ordering of timetables and bells, to the detailed regulation of bodily comportment, the body

is surrounded and constructed by technologies of power which serve
to organise, monitor, control and create it (Katz 1996).

Foucault's task in exploring such regimes is to create a history of
the different modes by which humans are made subjects. Three are of
special significance in this. The first are dividing practices, techniques
whereby different sorts of populations or categories of person are
created, by dividing them off from others. Such processes categorise,
separate, normalise and institutionalise populations. The isolation of
lepers, or the confinement of the poor or mad are examples of such
practices; and they are often given a physical or spatial expression
through separate buildings, different categories of ward, subdivisions
of the institution.

The second mode is through classificatory practices. The emergence of the social sciences in the nineteenth century allowed for the
creation of systems of knowledge through which individuals and
populations could be created and ordered. They both designated the
objects to be known – the individual and the population – and the
subjects – doctors, statisticians, demographers, behavioural experts,
sexologists – who had the authority to speak about them. Classificatory practices ordered mental diseases and allowed the separation of
the mad from the sane; provided taxonomies of the poor, distinguishing the deserving from the undeserving; and elaborated norms
of sexual behaviour, defining types of deviance.

Classificatory practices form part of the disciplining of populations. Through the appeal to collections of data and statistical
techniques, 'norms' are created against which individuals can be
judged and classified, and anomalous individuals or populations
made subject to corrective or therapeutic technologies. The context
in which such schemes of correction or therapy are elaborated and
applied is often an overtly humane one. Much of the history of
medicine or psychiatry, penal policy or treatment of the poor turns
around humanitarian reform. Part of Foucault's aim, however, is to
show how such progressive and enlightened responses are just as
much expressions of power as more overtly repressive ones. Foucault
overturns the progressive account given of medicine, or the treatment
of the insane, or the growth of sexual toleration and freedom, and
substitutes a darker account in which the development of the modern
age embodies not enlightenment and progress but new and different
forms of repression in which the disciplinary forces are not so much
external and physical, but internal and found in systems of thought
and the practices that support them.

The third mode is subjectification. This differs from the first two in that the focus is on active forms of self-formation in which individuals apply disciplinary techniques to themselves through technologies of the self. The extension of confession from its original religious context into wider secular forms of self-reflection and therapy provides one example; the control of the body through regimes of diet and exercise another. Often these processes of reflection, self-understanding and development are mediated by a specialist – a priest, a therapist, a personal trainer.

Power for Foucault operates at a covert and micro level. It is something that is diffused and disguised throughout the social system. This capillary character means that it is all pervasive, constitutive of social relations and practices. It is not so much exercised, as possessed, and it is embodied in the day-to-day practices of professionals such as doctors, psychologists, therapists, social workers. The disciplinary practices enjoined by such persons are the way in which the principles of carcereal society are institutionalised in everyday routines (Turner 1997).

Foucault did not directly address issues of the body in old age, but Katz and others have developed his insights in relation to the development of gerontological knowledge to show how old people have been constituted as the subjects of power/knowledge through the disciplines of gerontology and geriatrics (Katz 1996). Foucault showed how subjectivity was constructed at the level of the body and the population. This Katz argues is particularly relevant to older people since the aged body and the aged population in the form of demography have been the two special subjects of gerontological knowledge. Katz explores the processes whereby the aged have been defined as a population through technologies of differentiation such as almshouses, pension systems and social surveys. In the chapters that follow we will explore some of the implications for Foucault's perceptions for the treatment of the body in old age.

Work on the body has also been influenced by new theorising in relation to sexuality. Within feminism, the old distinction forged in the 1970s between sex and gender has been eroded, as sexuality and its bodily expression have come to be seen as no more natural and given than gender. Under the influence of Queer Theory, sexualities (the plural is significant) are increasingly perceived as socially constructed, constituted in and through discourse (Butler 1993). Such shifts also reflect the impact of the larger 'linguistic turn', whereby the focus of analysis has shifted from things and relationships to language and discourse. In such postmodern approaches the body is regarded wholly as a cultural construct, something that can only be apprehended through discourse and its related practices.

This radical epistemology has been subject to criticism both in relation to theorising about the body and more widely (Williams and Bendelow 1998). The social world may indeed be constituted in discourse, but this acts upon a physiological base that itself influences and structures that world. Discourse does not just fabricate bodies, bodies can also shape discourse and give us categories with which to think (a point we will return to in relation to the work of Mary Douglas). Within postmodernism, the body becomes oddly evanescent, and there is a sense of paradox that in focusing so much on the body as a social construct, we lose sight of the fundamental significance of embodiment. The critique of this radical epistemology has been particularly strong within gerontology where impairment, frailty and death have an undeniable reality (Bury, 1995, Williams and Bendelow 1998). Social constructionism and discourse analysis can be seen as having a heuristic quality to them, resting on a desire to see how far the approach can be pushed. But in the face of pain and death, such notions ultimately fall away.

The disembodied character of much writing about the body also relates to a second criticism, which concerns its overly theoretical character. Much of the early work in the field was highly theoretical, thus ironically reduplicating the tradition of abstraction and distance that it sought to criticise. Newer work has, however, begun to emerge that seeks to grasp the nature of social embodiment in a more concrete way, and collections edited by Davis (1997), Nettleton and Watson (1998), and Ellis and Dean (2000) have opened up fruitful new territories for analysis.

One of the few areas where an appreciation of the significance of the body in social life has always been present has been in anthropology; and the symbolic use of the body has been a central theme in anthropological work from Mauss (1934) to Firth (1973), Douglas (1966, 1970), Lévi-Strauss (1970, 1973, 1978) and Victor Turner (1969). Among earlier theorists, this emphasis had rested on the discredited idea that 'simple societies' were more bodily in nature, and that the body, its decoration and deployment in social life, was of greater significance; though it was also fuelled by the concern of anthropologists working in a structuralist mode to display the unity of culture and the structural congruencies between its different elements. Bringing these ideas across into the analysis of complex cultures soon revealed, however, the ways in which such symbolism of the body was central in western societies also, though masked by the earlier analytic traditions that emphasised the rational and the public as opposed to the bodily and day-to-day. The work of Mary Douglas was particularly influential in these developments, and we will discuss the relevance of her ideas more fully in Chapter 2. Norbert Elias's account of the Civilising Process (1978) whereby the body has been subject to a growing imposition of restraint through the internalisation of codes of conduct in relation to such aspects as eating, posture, bodily privacy, has been similarly influential in the historical sphere; and his ideas, as we shall see, have particular relevance to the meaning and history of bathing.

Another example of a theorist who dealt with the body before the sociology of the body had emerged is Erving Goffman (1961, 1969). Goffman was always sensitive to the ways bodies operated in the interactional order, and corporeal competence – for example how to negotiate one's way through a crowd – is central to his account of the world of social order. Goffman's people are always active agents, manipulators of meaning, and his account therefore acts as a welcome antidote to Foucauldian theorising in which the nexus of power/knowledge bears down oppressively on individuals and their bodies. His account of the micro-processes of the social world, particularly in relation to the institution and the role of inmates and custodians in it, has not been surpassed. He remains one of the supreme sociologists of the day-to-day, and thus of central importance to attempts to recast the analysis of community care nearer that level.

One of the most profound sources of influence on the discourses of the body in the twentieth century has been psychoanalysis. As a result of the work of Freud, it is now commonplace for us to see the bodily experiences of sex, birth, excretion as profoundly present in our lives. Though previously known to culture, it was largely so through the medium of jokes and other indecorous forms of comment; Freud brought this subterranean world into conscious review. Some of the themes of this book draw on these shared yet rarely acknowledged understandings. More recently, under the influence of post-structuralists like Lacan with their emphasis on language, Freud has come to be interpreted as less of a physiological reductionist, and analysis has shifted from the level of the biological to the symbolic. Culture imposes meanings on the anatomical parts; and the earlier focus on drives and instincts has been replaced by desire, the penis by the phallus. Though the imagery of the body remains central, it is now the body as constituted through language.

Finally, interest in the body has been fuelled by the perception that under conditions of high- or post-modernity, the body assumes a new significance in culture. The privatisation of meaning consequent on the decline of the religious world view produces a situation where people increasingly seek meaning at the individual, private level, and this includes in and through their bodies (Shilling 1993). The body, its exploration and development, become increasingly central in self identity; a project to be worked upon: managed, manipulated, controlled. This underwrites a range of phenomena from dieting, exercise, cosmetic surgery, alternative medicine and other regimes of well-being.

Shilling (1993) argues that our increasing capacity to control the body is accompanied by a crisis in its meaning. New reproductive techniques, organ transplants, high-tech interventions, cosmetic surgery erode the sense of what is natural for the body; and virtual reality raises radical questions about its existence and its links to identity. Culture explores these anxieties through the genre of Horror, or the current preoccupation in art with the body and its disintegration.

Within consumer culture the body is a vehicle for pleasure, display and self-expression. The creation of mass consumption in the twentieth century has gone with a re-orientation of the population away from the old virtues of thrift, hard work and sobriety and towards hedonistic enjoyment. Media and advertising have eroded the old restraints and promoted the new pleasures of purchase and consumption. Shopping has become a paradigm mode of modern society. With this has gone an extension of the commodity form into more and more of social life, including the experience of the body. Consumer culture is preoccupied with perfect bodies, spread through glamorised representations of advertising and the increasing dominance of the visual image in culture. Consumer culture promotes a vast range of body products, cosmetics, dietary aids, body maintenance publications. But the new body emphasis also contains strongly ascetic strands, representing anxiety and unease more than the pursuit of pleasure, and it often contains a strain of self punishment. Body techniques can involve denial, control, the assertion of dominance over the body in pursuit of the slim, toned physique that modern culture demands. Bordo (1993) presents dieting and muscle culture on a continuum, united against the common enemies of soft, unsolid, excessive flesh. They are panopticon technologies in which the body is monitored and controlled, and as such they need to be seen in the wider context of Foucault's disciplinary practices.

As Featherstone and Turner have commented, the reward for ascetic bodywork is no longer spiritual – as it was in the past with religious techniques of fasting and self-denial – but strongly material in the form of a more attractive, more marketable self (Featherstone 1991, Turner 1991) Health promotion despite its focus on health is heavily imbued with the values of consumer culture, the idealisation of youth and the body beautiful. Fitness and slimness are here associated with prudence, prescience and the other virtues of control and success. Much of the new culture of the body is about the denial of age and death. Featherstone comments on the particular threats to modern self identity posed by the existence of pictures and films that present the image of the person as they were in the past and in vivid contrast to how they are now, posing very directly to observer and individual the central mystery of aging. The sense of aging as a mask that obscures the real enduring features is an old one, but one that Featherstone argues is particularly threatening to modern identity. In the absence of a religious world view that can giving meaning to death, aging is simply failure; and the second half of life becomes a relentless set of exercises and practices to deny this.

Conclusion

In the chapters that follow, I will attempt to take forward a new analysis, applying insights from the sociology of the body to the field of community care. Bodies abound in social and health care, but this fact has not been foregrounded, for reasons that we have explored above. Focusing on bathing and washing enables us to take forward such an analysis, and from the perspective of both those who receive care and those who give it. Carework is bodywork and in the chapters that follow we will explore this dimension in the work. In doing this, I will also attempt to re-cast the level of analysis nearer the front line of care and the interactive processes wherein it is created. As we noted 'care' is a dynamic relationship that needs to be explored from both directions. Lastly, the book makes a plea for the significance of the quotidian and mundane. It is in such day-to-day rhythms that much of the meaning of people's lives lies, and we need to grasp this fact if we are to hope to understand the lives of older and disabled people and their careworkers. Without such an understanding, social policy fails to engage with the reality of its subject.

2 Cultures of bathing and the body in High Modernity

We are accustomed to viewing washing and bathing as essentially mundane actions, so obvious and ordinary that they require no explanation or analysis. They are part of corporeal existence that we take for granted and that exists at a level below articulation or thought. Though social life rests on such bodily activities, we ignore this in accounts of ourselves and wider society. Bodily life has indeed been something that has been progressively downplayed in the process of modernity, and to emphasise it in social life is to breach taboo: to risk vulgarity, to make a joke, to assert equality, or claim intimacy.

In this chapter, I will explore the history of washing and bathing in the West, and in the two very different cultures of ancient Rome and modern Japan. The purpose of this is to disturb our common-sense understandings of what these activities entail. Norms of cleanliness, habits of washing and bathing, have altered historically and varied cross culturally. The meaning of these practices is not fixed. We are, for example, used to treating bathing as a private, individual act, largely concerned with cleanliness and hygiene. But in other eras and cultures, bathing has had quite different connotations, and been linked to a diverse set of social practices, the meanings of which have varied greatly. In the chapter, we will explore some of this diversity, looking at, among other things, bathing as part of sociability, as a ritual of purification and separation, as a source of ancient virtue, as an element in competitive gentility and class conflict, as a medical treatment, a source of sensual pleasure, a means of unity with nature. Some of these elements still have resonance within modern practices. They are present, though largely in muted form. Others have disappeared; but their historical existence alerts us to the width of meanings that are potentially available. Lastly, in this chapter, we will explore the significance of bathing and washing as part of developments concerning the body in high modernity, exploring in particular modern ambivalence around the body, and the consequences of this for the experiences of disability and old age.

Bathing in antiquity

Bathing in the classical period was an essentially public, convivial activity in which the health of the body and the pleasure of the senses were united in an experience that was seen as both a necessity and a luxury. For Romans, the baths embodied the ideal of civic life. The public baths of a city were a source of pride. Often a gift from a wealthy citizen or the emperor, their closure could be used as a punishment for rebellious cities. The baths were public spaces, places of resort, where citizens shared publicly in bodily processes. They thus endorsed a certain egality of the body; and emperors sometimes made a point of attending the public baths in the attempt to promote the idea of a united and classless society (Yegül 1992). Attending the baths was part of the day-to-day pattern of life of most Roman citizens. Work started at daybreak and continued to noon, when business finished and men would customarily repair to the baths for several hours. People rarely bathed in the evening, at night or in the morning; so although baths were used to mark transitions, they were not the transitions that are customary today. Men and women ordinarily bathed apart, usually by means of different hours, or sometimes separate rooms. After undressing, the bather would undertake exercise. In the classical system, this could be either natural or violent. Violent or muscular exercise involved activities like running, wrestling, active sports or moving the limbs in prescribed ways. Milder forms were also popular: ball games for men, hoop rolling for women. Natural exercise involved the exercise of the mind or senses in reading, discussing, talking, singing. Swimming, though well regarded as an exercise, was not a primary activity at the baths and mostly took place in rivers or the sea. The unheated pools at the baths were mainly used for wading and splashing. Exercise was followed by what was regarded as the best part of the experience, the hot baths, a series of rooms with progressively greater heat, followed by a cold plunge. Heat epitomised luxury for the Romans, and the hotter the baths the more luxurious. At various points aromatic oils could be used to cleanse and massage the body.

Exercise in the classical period thus entailed both the mind and the body, and was linked to wider concepts of well-being. The harmony of mind and body was an important element in classical therapeutics, and underpinned the Greek ideal of the gymnasium. Medicine in the classical period was predominantly preventive, aiming to treat and maintain the healthy body; and diet and exercise were its main therapies. The baths were also regarded as restorative and therapeutic, and regular attendance part of maintaining or recovering good health. Health and well being were closely linked in this system of ideas.

The baths were also places of sensory delight, where people could enjoy the pleasures of light and space, being in large well-lit rooms, looking up into the airy vault, seeing the costly marble, the play of light on water. They were sociable places where one could meet friends. Much drinking and talking took place there; and dinner after the baths was regarded as the most pleasing way to end the day. Other pleasures were also available. Female and male prostitutes could be found, and a private bath with a prostitute could be arranged as a preliminary to sex. Attacks on the luxury of the baths focused on the encouragement they gave to effeteness and vice.

Turkish baths are the direct descendants of the classical baths transmitted via Byzantium and the culture of Islam, though with significant differences (Kilito 1993). In the *hammam*, the process of bathing became less elaborated, the experience more tranquil and the level of light lower. With the exception of mineral spas, there was no longer a communal bathing pool, and people bathed separately using basins. The loss of the culture of exercise is a particularly significant difference. Attendance became weekly.

Baths in the Roman world were thus located in series of discourses: of pleasure and luxury, of health and well being, of personal and social cultivation. Many of the elements that made up the experience we still recognise today, but not always in these combinations or with these meanings. For example, baths and showers can often be used to mark out the transitions of the day including, as for the Romans, between the world of work and of leisure. The enjoyment of relaxation and hot water is a common experience, though one that is now seen as a private activity. Other elements have separated themselves off into specialist activities performed in different settings, though sometimes still called 'baths'. Swimming baths encompass some of the elements of the classical tradition: the pleasure of being in the water, the sociability, the sense of light and space; and the architecture sometimes consciously echoes that of the classical era. Other elements of the experience, however, such as eating and drinking, now take place in quite different settings.

Massage parlours share some of the erotic connotations of the baths, but again located in a different context. The therapeutic significance of baths has become much more muted as modern medicine has abandoned the old focus on regimens of good health, leaving interventions of that sort to the burgeoning territory of alternative medicine and the linked area of the beauty/therapy/health complex. The growing popularity of modern health spas, with their mixture of beauty treatments, stress reduction and the pursuit of well being, is part of this.

Bathing in Japan

Bathing has a long history in Japan. Traditionally communal, the wooden tub filled with hot water formed the centre of family and neighbourly life in the village. By the Tokugawa or Edo period, public bathhouses were common in urban areas, and they are often depicted in the prints of the 'floating world'. Offering both hot plunge and steam baths, they were mostly frequented by men, with female attendants who sometimes acted as entertainers or prostitutes. In the Meiji period, public bathhouses became used by a wider section of the population. Today they are mainly found in traditional areas of the city. There are separate entrances for men and women, with children moving freely between the two sections (mixed bathing is uncommon now and mainly confined to hot springs). The dressing area is often decorated in a traditional Japanese style, with the bathing area bright and tiled, how the Japanese think of the West. Washing takes place before entering the bath. The water is kept at a temperature of 47 degrees, and plentiful hot water is associated with luxury and wealth (Clark 1994).

Though public bath houses are still being built, their number is in dramatic decline (a drop of 40 per cent between 1965–85), and they are mostly to be found in poorer areas and used by older people who value sociability. Post-war affluence has killed off the habit of public bathing as the majority of Japanese now have baths in their own homes. In the post-war period, the domestic bath became one of the emblems of economic success (by 1968, 65 per cent of households had a bath at home). This shift away from communal bathing has provoked academic and public laments in which the traditional community-oriented values of Japan are seen as giving way to western individualism. Clark agrees that bathing is now a more private experience than it was in the past. Bathing however remains a cultural marker of Japaneseness. In the debates within Japan about modernity and westernisation, bathing belongs very clearly to that part of life that falls on the Japanese as opposed to the western side.

Within families, bathing takes place in the evening after the man of the house has returned from work. Hot baths are particularly valued as a means of washing away the stresses of the day as a 'salaryman'. Women are responsible for drawing the bath which, like the evening meal, forms part of the daily routine of the household. Traditionally families bathed in strict order, with the men going first by age, followed by the women by age. Clark notes that though this 'bathing order' is widely recognised, the reality is more flexible. Washing is a separate activity from bathing, and takes place prior to getting into the tub, sometimes in a slightly different space and using a shower head. Despite strong American influences in the post-war era and limited living space, the Japanese have remained resistant to showers.

Many Japanese aspire to larger baths that would hold more people. Japanese couples and young families often bath together, and the bond that develops as a result of such skin-to-skin contact in the warm water is valued and given a special term: 'skinship'. Bathing together is associated with confidences and emotional closeness. Fathers share in this intimate bond with their children, though the long hours of the 'salaryman' threaten this. By their teen years, children bath alone or with the parent of the same sex, though it is customary to bathe as a family at the hot springs.

Bathing in Japan can also draw on Buddhist or Taoist influenced ideas concerning unity with the beauty of nature. One of the pleasures of the hot springs consists in being able to lie in water while enjoying the trees and rocks that surround the pools and baths. In the past, portable baths were available that could be put up as part of pleasure excursions to view blossom or snow; to be able to do this while in the water offered an additional refinement to the experience. In a recent photographic celebration of bathing there is a striking photo sequence in which a glazed cable car containing ten small bath tubs filled with water and occupied by Japanese men is transported across a coastal scenery of beautiful rocks and waves (Koren 1996). The nearest we come in the West to such ideas are as an aspect of nineteenth-century nature cure, particularly in Germany where showers and 'light and air baths' (together with 'sun baths') taken in the woods in direct contact with nature formed part of regimes of therapy and well being.

Bathing is an act of immersing oneself in symbols; and Scott locates it in the context of a series of symbolic oppositions in

Japanese culture concerning pure/impure, inside/outside, up/down in which the transitions into the home and between states are accompanied by acts of cleansing that draw on Shinto concepts of pollution and purification. Japanese people wash their hands on entering the home (as they do a Shinto shrine) and sometimes gargle. The explanation that is given of this by participants is˜ in terms of washing away the germs of the city, and daily bathing is not perceived by the Japanese as having anything to do with religion. Scott however believes that cleanliness and purity of body and soul are intertwined in Japan in such a way that the daily bath is experienced as a profound process of renewal. Baths are traditionally associated with the rituals of the life cycle and with important events, such as going to war or the end of the year both of which were traditionally accompanied by bathing; and this again underlines their symbolic significance.

Natural symbols, rites of passage and coercive cultures

Washing and bathing are enduring features of bodily practice and, as such, classic examples of 'natural symbols' in the sense outlined by Mary Douglas (1970). Douglas argues that while symbols have to be interpreted in the context of particular social and cultural configurations, so that there are no pan-cultural or pan-historical symbolic meanings, certain objects and relationships are so recurring in human experience that they present natural material for the creation of symbolic meaning. The body is the prime example of this; and the processes of birth, death and physiological life offer potent material for incorporation within symbolic systems. Washing and bathing frequently feature as part of this repertoire. Water is a long-established natural symbol of purification and cleansing, and its use runs through religious and ritual practice. Washing the hands before praying, for example, is found in Hindu, Muslim and other traditions. Sources of pure water such as springs are often associated with shrines and places of religious pilgrimage. Some at least of the spa and watering places that developed in a secular context in the seventeenth and eighteenth centuries in Britain had had earlier existences as holy wells and places of religious healing. Even secular settings like modern spas and health farms retain some of this quasi-religious character in their use of the language of purification and renewal.

Baths often feature as part of rites of passage where they are used to denote transitions between social states. The term originates with van Gennep and has been elaborated by Victor Turner as part of a wider analysis of marginality and anti-structure (van Gennep 1908, V. W. Turner 1969). Rites of passage classically have a tripartite structure: separation, transition, incorporation. Christian baptism offers one of the clearest examples of the use of water as a symbol of transition and renewal, in which through the pouring on of water the baby makes the passage from physiological birth to social birth, and depending on theological position from a state of original sin to one of conditional grace. The symbolism of water and of the bath is most strongly present in those traditions that use total immersion, where the rite marks the transition, typically of an adult, from a worldly state to one of incorporation into the body of the faithful, the passage through the deep water symbolising the passage through death to the new life beyond.

Rites of passage using baths are also found in secular settings, though their operation often remains hidden and unacknowledged. For example people are frequently given a bath as part of the transition into institutions. Prisoners are made to bath as part of their admission into prison; baths are commonly given to old people when admitted to a ward; even patients entering psychiatric facilities are sometimes bathed (Goffman 1961, Littlewood 1991, Fitzgerald and Sim 1979). In so far as explanation of such practices is given, it is in terms of hygiene, offering another example, as Douglas (1966) has argued in relation to rationalistic explanations of Jewish food avoidances, of the ways in which modern society uses hygiene and 'science' to explain and justify what are essentially social and symbolic concerns. Bathing and showering here mark social transitions, and have little to do with health or hygiene. Sometimes these baths are accompanied by other bodily practices that have a similar quality to them, such as cutting hair or imposing uniforms. Prison haircuts are traditionally short and harsh, and explanations for this are sometimes given in terms of concern with cleanliness and lice. Similarly Primo Levi (1987) found on entry to the concentration camp, new inmates were showered. Explanations in terms of health or hygiene of inmates make no sense in this context, and their use – together with techniques like shaving the head and confiscating clothes – point to the ways in which bathing and showering can represent techniques of coercion as well as transition.

These rituals of – literally – de-gradation are part of the proc-esses that produce Foucault's docile bodies. Recurring through the history and symbolism of bathing is a cruel, coercive streak. This is most obviously so in relation to prisons, hospitals and especially mental asylums. Water had been used in the treatment of the mentally ill from the seventeenth century. Though earlier forms of water treatment were based on the rationale of shocking the patient back into the sanity he/she had lost (Scull 1993), it is hard to avoid the sense of sadism present in such practices. Immersion in cold water was widely used to subdue and shock mental patients, and the habit of 'packing' in which patients were wrapped very tightly in wet bindings continued well into the twentieth century. Baths are part of coercive cultures, and something of this is nearly always present where someone *is* bathed. Power is exercised over their bodies which are required to be exposed and immersed in circumstances where they are naked and the administrator is not. These coercive uses of water also often impose humiliating postures and situations.

The use of machinery represents a further objectification. Histories of bathing and washing, particularly those that emphasise the development of sanitary machinery and equipment, often have a slightly bizarre, surrealist quality to them, and this is true of Siegfried Giedion's classic and pioneering account of 1948 *Mechanization Takes Command*. Giedion's theme is the imposition of mechanisation in modern life, and bathing and washing illustrate the ways in which this takes place in relation to the bodies of men and women. His account is influenced by Surrealism and the work of Max Ernst with its use of nineteenth-century trade engravings of baths and bathing equipment, full of drains and plugs, douches and showers, straps and taps. Such equipment reinforces the objectification that is always in play when someone *is* bathed and we will explore this further in subsequent chapters when we explore the significance of baths in day centres. Equipment both distances the person from direct human contact, putting a barrier between them and the operator, and acts to objectify them by providing the means whereby they are trapped, caged, made subject to the machine. Echoes of this remain even where, as in relation to community care, the context is largely a benign one.

Elias and changing concepts of washing and bathing in the West

We now turn to the history of bathing as it emerged in the West. Norbert Elias in *The Civilizing Process* argues that we have witnessed a major shift in sensibility concerning the management of the body since the middle ages, and he describes this in terms of the diffusion of codes of conduct developed in courtly society to the population as a whole (Elias 1978). Through a study of the changing content of books of manners, he charts the gradual imposition of restraint over the body and its expression across a number of dimensions: eating, sleeping, sexual, eliminatory, emotional. In this the thresholds of shame, disgust and repugnance are raised, so that conduct that was once ordinary becomes increasingly distasteful. This imposition of restraint is accompanied by a growing individualisation of the body and the self. In relation to food, for example, Elias charts the shift from the habit of eating from a common dish with fingers, through the arrival of the fork, to an expectation of individual plates and glasses; in relation to sleeping arrangements, the shift from the acceptability of shared beds with the same sex to the expectation that individuals will sleep alone (unless with a sexual partner). There are a similar impositions of constraint over nakedness (the arrival of clothes for night, the abandonment of mixed nude bathing); over spitting and blowing the nose on clothes (the arrival of the handkerchief); over defecating and urinating in public. As with sex, these bodily functions were increasingly moved behind the screens of domestic life, into separate and private spaces, where their existence becomes something that cannot be remarked upon in polite company. The new codes of restraint extended to the emotions. Violent fluctuations of mood and feeling that Elias regards as characteristic of the medieval psyche, together with a 'primitive' delight in acts of cruelty and violence, become increasingly unacceptable. The animal origins of meat, in the form of joints, heads, or whole part of beasts and an accompanying relish in offal, are increasingly played down.

For Elias what is important about these shifts is the way in which they are internalised and naturalised, so that what has to be described and explained in some detail in the conduct books of the sixteenth century before it can be condemned, becomes so obvious and assumed in later ages that it scarcely needs to be mentioned. Whole dimensions of life are thus removed from the conscious review and comment of civilised people. In the modern period, as self restraint becomes second nature, overt social rules and sanctions are less significant and a more relaxed demeanour in the twentieth century becomes possible, because it rests on a bedrock of internalised self control.

The history of washing and bathing parallels these processes. Baths existed in the medieval period, though they were not connected with cleanliness but with pleasure and conviviality (Vigarello 1988).

Baths for the wealthy were one of a number of sensual pleasures associated with feasting, luxury and making love. For ordinary people there were public bath and steam houses which were associated with gambling, drinking, and a certain amount of impropriety. Men and women bathed naked and together. By the late middle ages, however, the new thresholds of decency meant that mixed bathing was increasing disapproved of. Public bathhouses came to be perceived as disorderly places, and from the late middle ages were increasingly shut down by the public authorities. Among the wealthy too, bathing fell into disuse, but for different reasons concerning new perceptions of water.

During the early modern period, a major shift occurred in the evaluation of water which came to be perceived as dangerous to the body. Skin was regarded as porous; and water, especially hot water, was believed to penetrate the body and weaken its vital fluids. Young children were no longer bathed in water since its action would prolong the softness of a system that was already too moist; the process of growing up was seen as a process of drying out. Baths came to be seen as threatening to the system, something that debilitated the body and sapped its strength. They became things of trepidation, only be embarked upon with caution, and ideally under medical supervision; it became advisable to rest for some time after a bath and to avoid going too soon into the air.

Washing in the early modern period was a similarly circumscribed activity. Only the face and hands were washed with water. Body smells among the refined were reduced by frequent changes of linen which removed sweat and other effluvia from the skin, by techniques of 'dry washing' such as rubbing down with white cloths or brushes, or by wiping down with perfumes and spirits. Perfumes were not simply used to mask smells but believed to have active properties, purifying corrupt air and fortifying and strengthening the body. Water on the head was particularly dangerous, and hair was cleaned by rubbing with bran.

Washing was less a matter of hygiene than of decency, the wish to avoid appearing clownish and ill bred in good company. Etiquette books of the medieval and early modern period emphasise the cleanliness of only the visible parts of the body: the face and hands. Pages were taught to wash these as part of seigneural conduct, and offering water to wash hands was a mark of courtesy. By the sixteenth century, however, new demands of cleanliness were being made in relation to linen. In the middle ages few people had had much linen and it was mostly hidden under the sumptuous clothes that were the main focus of display. In the early modern period, linen becomes an increasingly prominent and visible aspect of dress. Displaying fresh white linen becomes a mark of gentility. Etiquette books emphasise the importance of frequent change of linen; and the cycle of shirt changing speeds up through the sixteenth, seventeenth and eighteenth centuries as expectations rise. Vigarello argues that this emphasis on linen represents a new sensibility in which concern with cleanliness has penetrated below the immediate surface of clothes, but has as yet stopped short of the body itself. Clean linen allowed the body to be 'imagined' in a new way, but one that stopped short of the thorough-going surveillance that characterises modern concerns with bathing and showering. Cleanliness in this period is still an aspect of manners, something that is visible, superficial and social rather than concerned with the state of the body itself.

In the eighteenth century the practice of bathing begins to reappear among the upper classes. Bath houses and cold water plunges are common features in eighteenth-century landscapes (examples can be seen at Rousham, Kedleston, Walton, Painswick). Spas and watering places became increasingly popular, and plunge baths are among the facilities they offered (Hembry 1990, 1997). This new enthusiasm for bathing was however located in the context of a different structure of ideas. Water, particularly cold water, was now the bearer of virtue. Cold plunges were believed to harden and strengthen the body, cold water was now associated with classical virtue, promoting moral as well as physical vigour. This cold water was an austere substance promoting Republican virtues. The ancients were thought to have bathed in cold water, and proponents of cold baths, like Sir John Floyer, linked them to the Roman virtues of stoicism and strength, contrasting this with the soft languors of modern decadence (Floyer 1706).

In the French context, Vigarello locates similar developments in the late eighteenth century, and linked to Rousseauesque ideas of 'natural' childbirth, breast feeding, lighter classical clothes. Emile was brought up to bathe in cold water (Rousseau 1764: 59). Washing and cold water are now associated with simplicity and nature, and with the freshness of the Romantic vision. In the politics of the body, cleanliness is now linked to natural virtue, and set in opposition to the vain affectation and artifice of aristocratic culture with its powder and pomade. As yet the opposition is not with the dirtiness of the poor. The stage is thus set for the development of the new bourgeois standard of cleanliness in which the whole body becomes the focus of concern.

The spread of the new bourgeois standard

The new standard of cleanliness that emerged in the early nineteenth century was driven by social preoccupations in the form of the competitive pursuit of gentility and personal refinement. Cleanliness from the mid-nineteenth century becomes a mark of social and spiritual superiority, and an emblem in the war between the classes. Moral purity was increasingly equated with physical purity. Though the phrase 'cleanliness is next to godliness' was used by Wesley in the eighteenth century, it is only in the nineteenth that it achieves prominence, linked to a wider set of virtues around temperance and self control. Frequent washing and bathing come to be associated with the bourgeois culture of self-discipline, and find their parallel in attitudes to sexuality, work and money (Wilkie 1986). Cold baths in particular become associated with the control of male sexual desire, dampening down 'overheated' sexual drives. In the late nineteenth century growing anxieties about masturbation resulted in the popularisation of cold bathing and showering as part of the public school regime.

The new structure of ideas concerning washing and bathing emerged in Britain and America. From the 1850s onwards, regular personal washing becomes part of the routine of middle-class Americans (Bushman and Bushman 1988). Sullivan's luxury hotel built for the Chicago World Fair of 1893 failed because it did not have ensuite bathrooms. By 1900 bathrooms were standard in middle-class American homes. By the 1920s 'decent' people in Middletown (Muncie) regarded a second bathroom as desirable. For the working class in the US a bathroom was standard in new housing after the First World War. The Lynds in Middletown noted that 25 per cent of working-class dwellings 'lacked' such facilities, though the word was itself indicative of new expectations (Wilkie 1986). By the time of the New Deal, official housing standards required a bathroom (Williams 1991). In Britain the pattern was similar though the spread was slower. Even as late as 1873, the aristocratic Carlton Towers was rebuilt without a single bathroom, though by 1881, the houses in Bedford Park, aimed at upper-middle-class people of 'artistic' sensibilities, were advertised as all having bathrooms (Swenarton 1977, Girouard 1979, Laing and Laing nd).

The spread of the new standard was assisted by technological advances, such as the development of the fixed self-emptying bathtub, the provision of clean piped water and easier and cheaper means to heat it (Wright 1960, Daunton 1983, Wilkie 1986, Goubert 1986). These together created the new defined space of the 'bath room' (previously washing and bathing had taken place on a temporary basis in the bedroom). Hot water also made possible the use of soap on the body. In the eighteenth century most soap was harsh, tallow-based and primarily used to wash clothes – getting clean was mainly about getting your clothes clean, and people rinsed their hands without using soap. Olive oil based 'cosmetic' soaps were available for the wealthy, but as their name implies they were primarily seen as beauty treatments sold by perfumiers, and taxed as luxury goods (Bushman and Bushman 1988). It was only after the 1880s that new soaps became widely available based on palm oil that could be used on both clothes and persons. (Imperial Leather and Palmolive are examples of this new generation of widely promoted soaps.)

Bathrooms in homes were not the only facilities supporting the new code: and public baths also provided means of washing and bathing. The public bath movement had its origins in England in the 1830s and 1840s, spreading to continental Europe and America (Williams 1991, Bird 1995). The first public baths built in England at public expense was the St George's Bath (1828) in Liverpool (a city which pioneered popular provision). In 1846 the Public Baths and Washhouses Act empowered parishes to provide local facilities; and by 1896, 200 municipalities in England had public baths. In Germany and America large elaborate bathing facilities became a source of municipal pride. In France the focus was more on laundry provision. Larger public baths typically contained a variety of facilities: swimming pools, bath tubs, steam and air baths, as well as facilities for washing and ironing clothes and bed linen. American and German public 'baths' were almost always in the form of showers, contrasting with the British tradition of tubs.

Public baths need to be set in the context of a series of municipal reforms promoted in response to the new conditions of the great cities. Like clean water, sewerage, public lighting and town gas, they reflect changing ideas about the roles and duties of urban government. Public health measures were in large part driven by fear of diseases, particularly cholera, emanating from the poor, and the provision of public baths was an attempt to raise standards of cleanliness – and morality – among the working class. During the nineteenth century, however, public baths were also used by the middle class in the – as yet not uncommon – absence of a private bathroom. An amendment to the 1846 Act laid down that separate baths should be provided for the middle and working classes. The First Class baths charged more and were intended to subsidise other provision.

In the early twentieth century, the accent shifted away from washing towards swimming. Public baths were increasingly built in conjunction with libraries and public halls, on prominent sites with imposing architecture; and they lost the earlier focus on personal cleaning. Swimming was encouraged as a means of improving the health of the nation, especially building up the poor physiques of working class men revealed in the Boer War recruitment, and it joined other competitive sports developed and codified in Britain in this era (Laing and Laing nd). The different functions were increasingly separated out, and by the mid twentieth century, these 'baths' were largely about leisure and sport rather than cleanliness.

This plurality of purposes and meanings is reflected in the language of bathing and the ambiguity that still attaches to the pronunciation of bath, for it is only in certain grammatical forms that the difference between 'bath' and 'bathe' is made clear. 'Bathe' is used in relation to swimming, though perhaps through its echoes of lave, also has poetical and mythical connotations that endow it with a more refined and dignified tone. 'Bath' is down to earth, and more closely linked with getting clean. The meanings of bathing are, however, wider than this and the survival of the two pronunciations indicates something of this.

The gospel of germs and the modern concern with hygiene

As we have seen, cleanliness in the earlier nineteenth century was primarily about gentility not hygiene in the sense of concern with disease. But in the period 1890 to 1930 the popularisation of germ theory and its translation into day-to-day practices in the home meant that washing and cleaning assumed a new importance in the war against germs (Tomes 1998). Germ theory presented a new scientific account of infection, but one Tomes argues that was able to build on elements of the earlier sanitary science that had presented the causes of infection as lying in contaminated water, miasmas and human filth. Though opposed scientifically, the two sets of ideas both endorsed health practices focused on the household, supporting a growing preoccupation with plumbing, ventilation and the removal of dirt. The gospel of germs was taken up and promoted especially in the US by Progressive Era institutions like the Boy Scouts, YMCA, anti-TB associations, though the chief target of its propaganda was housewives. The new understanding of germ theory led to changes in food handling – for example, not leaving food uncovered – as well as in the increased emphasis on the use of handkerchiefs and avoiding open coughing and spitting. The discovery that tuberculoisis was not an illness of constitution but of transmission was particularly important, and the crusade against TB became a major popular health movement promoting the gospel of germs. Facial hair came to be seen as insanitary, and kissing babies was discouraged. There were new concerns with separate and individual provision, for example, removing the common cup from drinking fountains, and providing separate cakes of soap in hotels. Germ theory thus promoted greater separation and individuation in bodily practices than had been current before. Casual physical contact came to be seen as potentially contaminating in a new way. Crowded trains, public lavatories, door handles, all came to be seen as a potential source of disease. Germ theory provided the scientific rationale for processes of separation and distance that were underway at a deeper level within society.

These developments in relation to popular hygiene laid the foundation for twentieth-century modernism, as the elaborate dusty and dark furnishings of the Victorian interior gave way to a stripped-down aesthetic of clean, wipeable surfaces and pale colours. Theorists of the Modern Movement in architecture repeatedly used the term 'clean' in their writings; and TB sanatoria, with their bare white walls, sun filled, open air balconies, became one of the emblematic building types of modern architecture (examples include Aalto's Paimio sanatorium, Duiker's Zonnestraal). Developments in the bathroom reflected these shifts. Bathrooms when they originally emerged in the mid-nineteenth century were decorated on the same lines as the rest of the house, often modelled on the dressing room with heavy, built-in mahogany fitments. But as the new concern with hygiene grew, bathrooms became increasingly minimal in their decoration. China ware was no longer decorated but pure white, and designed to minimise dust. Rugs and carpets were removed and replaced by mats and wipeable flooring. Obscured glass replaced heavy curtains. By the 1930s, bathroom chairs were white with cork seats, again to minimise dust and germs. Wall-tiled bathrooms were one of the attractions of the speculative built semis of the era (Swenarton 1977). The bathroom had emerged as a specialised space in the house, with its own differentiated furniture and decor.

Discourses of class and national superiority

During the nineteenth and early twentieth centuries, questions of washing, bathing and personal smell came to be deployed in a discourse of class superiority and distance. As the middle class adopted the new standard in hygiene, a social gulf opened between them and the working class in terms of personal habits and smell. Eighteenth century interest in how people smelt turned around the effects of diet and climate (Corbin 1986); but increasingly in the nineteenth century bourgeois perceptions came to focus on the smell of the poor. Thackeray wrote of the Great Unwashed, and American writers of the period referred to 'tenement odor' (Thackeray 1848, Laing and Laing nd.). Bourgeois imagery of the masses begins to construct them in terms of filth: the stench of the poor, their fetid, animal existence in the dark spaces of the city. This excremental imagery in part arises out of the concerns of the sanitary reformers, but it also reflects changes in class relations. The rise of the great cities both intensified social contact and produced a new emphasis on social differentiation and separation, exemplified in the geographical zoning of the city in class terms. In this, issues around dirt and the capacity to clean oneself came to mark out social distance; cleanliness and smell became part of a repertoire of gestures of separation and classification underwriting the wider social order. Smell entered the world of class conflict.

The perception that the poor smelt continued into the interwar period. Somerset Maugham wrote in 1922:

> I do not blame the working man because he stinks, but stink he does. It makes social intercourse difficult for persons of a sensitive nostril. The matitudinal tub divides the classes more effectively than birth, wealth or education.
>
> (Maugham 1922, p142)

Orwell concurred:

> The real secret of class distinctions in the West ... is summed up in the four frightful words which people are chary of uttering, but which were banded about quite freely in my childhood. *The lower classes smell.*
>
> (Orwell 1937, p112)

'Coals in the bath' remained a common middle class sneer throughout the period (Swenarton 1977).

In America, although the gospel of germs rested on concepts of the chain of disease that linked the classes and supported public health interventions for the poor, it also underwrote a new social separation. The poor in the American cities or the rural south could afford none of the basics of the new hygiene practices: clean running water, baths, and safe milk. Increasingly the middle class associated poor, immigrant and non-white populations with dirt, disease and germs, deepening divisions of class and race, and providing a rationale that was used to support segregation (Tomes 1998).

Baths and washing are also embedded in discourses of national superiority that reflect both material progress and cultural difference. In the nineteenth century, England pioneered the provision of clean water, sewage disposal and the public health measures that supported the new emphasis on cleanliness (Goubert 1989); and these advances in urban planning were carried forward energetically in the United States, so that by the end of the century, Anglo-Saxon plumbing had become a byword for efficiency and high standards. Britain and America were both centres for the development and production of sanitary ware. In the American mind, cleanliness and bathing came to be associated with social and cultural superiority (Wilkie 1986). America was seen as more 'ahead' in this, as in other spheres, and American standards of hygiene were contrasted with the dirtier habits of Europeans. Promoting public baths was seen as one of the ways of encouraging the Americanisation of immigrants (Williams 1991).

It is true that in France the new gospel of cleanliness did indeed make slower progress. Bathrooms were still a comparative rarity in bourgeois homes in the early years of the twentieth century, and were largely associated in the French mind with tourist hotels and luxury brothels (Goubert 1989, Corbin 1986). Baths still required a therapeutic justification; and most French doctors remained distrustful of the immoderate use of water. The habit of bathing or showering regularly remained uncommon into the post-war era. In 1962 only 29 per cent of French households had a bath or shower (Nirascou 1998). In 1951 *Elle* ran a notorious article in which French habits were held up unfavourably against American standards (Ross 1995). This was the period in which the French economy and culture were about to undergo rapid modernisation, and the article struck a chord in debates about modernisation and economic affluence. Despite economic developments that have placed France above Britain in economic terms, patterns of difference persist. A survey reported in *Le Figaro* in 1998 suggested that only 47 per cent of the French take a daily bath or shower. In Britain and Germany, the figure was 70 per cent. Soap consumption varied in proportion (1400g per person per year in GB and 600g in France) suggesting that the figures do not simply reflect differences in reporting (Nirascou 1998).

Corbin, writing from a French perspective, argues that attitudes to cleanliness and smell cannot simply be seen in terms of economic development. Reflecting on the historical data he concludes:

> The relative indifference shown by the French to cleanliness, their rejection of water, their long tolerance of strong bodily odours, and their continued privatisation of excrement and rubbish cannot be explained solely by a secret distrust of innovation, by relative poverty, or by slow urbanisation. It was the collective attitude towards the body, the organic functions, and the sensory messages that governed behaviour.
>
> (Corbin 1986: 173)

In this, French cultural attitudes are implicitly contrasted with Anglo-Saxon puritanism. Kira writing from an American perspective in the 1960s, noted how Europeans were 'highly amused over our concern – nay preoccupation – with body odors which they regard as 'perfectly natural" '(1967: 15).

National differences are here embedded in two rival discourses of superiority. One is about material advance in which the degree of involvement with the new culture of cleanliness is a marker of economic development. This operates at both the simple level of material goods – the social wealth necessary to produce fast showers, high quality fitments, abundant clean water, in parallel with other consumption goods – and at the associated level of cultural attitudes that arise from such material advance – the expectations that support the new practices of washing. These economic realities create a discourse of national superiority in which grubbiness, body smells and poor facilities represent cultural backwardness.

The second counter discourse regards such preoccupations with cleanliness and washing as puritanical and body hating, arising from a fear of the body and its natural odours. From the French perspective, concern with cleanliness and germs is regarded as part of American obsessionalism. Although these differences are played out in terms of national rivalries, particularly in relation to the cultural wars of the French against Anglo-Saxon influence, they in fact reflect tensions within modernity that are more general. We turn to these in the next section.

The intensification of themes around washing in the post-war era

As we have seen, the nineteenth-century bourgeois code extended the gaze of cleanliness from just the visible parts on the surface to the whole body. During the post-war era this process continued and intensified, and a new standard of cleanliness was increasingly exacted from all. The old class-based discourse around smell fell into disuse, and baths became commonplace in working-class homes in the post-war era, though the high cost of heating water meant that their use was limited and they remained weekly events for most working-class families well into the late twentieth century. The 1970s and 1980s were a turning point in personal habits, and frequent baths or showers became the norm for large parts of British society. Increasingly smell has become associated not with class but inadequacy. Social workers use smell as a indicator of families that are not managing; and the old class discourse of smell has thus become residualised in the persons of the underclass.

The growing focus on the body as a whole was also reflected in cosmetics and bathroom goods. In the 1950s creams and cosmetics for women focused on the face: powder, lipstick, face creams, toners. The main site for intervention was the face, and though women also aimed to have attractive figures, these could in part be achieved by underwear that moulded and concealed the body. By the 1980s however this was no longer good enough and bodies had to be dieted, toned and exercised into the required shape. Control was thus extended to the whole body and internalised. A parallel development occurred in relation to creams and lotions. The 1980s saw a massive expansion in the range of these products aimed at the body as a whole: shower gels, body lotions, all-over moisturisers, exfolients, anti-cellulite creams (cellulite as a 'problem' was invented in the 1980s). In part this represents a growing elaboration of the market consequent on rising incomes, but it also reflects new demands being made on the body and its presentation.

Changes in the bathroom also reflect this intensification of concern. As the frequency of bathing and showering rises, so too does demand on bathroom space. From the 1980s it becomes common for larger houses to feature multiple bathrooms; and in expensive housing, the ratio of bathrooms to bedrooms now approaches one to one. Bathrooms are also becoming increasingly personal space. People appear to be more unwilling to share communal facilities. Wiles's study of women's preferences for private as opposed to NHS hospital care found that not having to share a bathroom or toilet was an important factor for respondents (Wiles 1993); and hotel bedrooms of even a modest character now have en-suite facilities. Gurney (1998), Chapman and Lucas (1998) all argue that expectations of levels of privacy around washing, bathing and excreting are increasing. New guidelines issued to schools, for example, by the Department of Education and Employment state that communal showers are no longer acceptable (*Guardian* 21.12.99). The meaning of the bathroom is also shifting. No longer just the small utilitarian spaces of the past, these new bathrooms are increasingly presented as places of luxury and bodily pleasure. In the imagery of house sale promotions, there is a clear eroticisation of the en-suite bathroom attached to the master bedroom (Chapman and Lucas 1998). This has sometimes gone with a new 'zen' emphasis on bathing – candles, music – as a source of individual pleasure and a form of spiritual escape from the stresses of the modern world.

The rival discourses of baths and showers

Cultural shifts in relation to the body are also reflected in the growing popularity of showers. Showers developed in the nineteenth century out of what had been termed rain baths (largely used for hydrotherapy treatments) and, though commonly used in America and parts of Continental Europe, remained relatively unusual in Britain until the 1970s when there was a rapid expansion in installation (in 1975 only 11 per cent of dwellings had a shower; in 1985, 40 per cent) (Business and Research Associates 1986). Most of these showers remain in the relatively ineffective form of a shower over the bath, and few have the pump action needed if there is to be any force to the water. Showers in Britain thus remain a secondary form, but one that is more popular with the young and men. This pattern of uptake reflects the different 'discourses' of baths and showers.

Showers are located in a discourse of youth, energy, vigour, modernity. The action of the water, particularly in a power shower, acts like a massage, pounding the skin and invigorating the body. Showers are regarded as time saving. There is an immediacy in the way that the water is delivered – you slam on a shower – that chimes with modern preoccupations with speed, efficiency and get-up-and-go. They reflect a culture of impatient and I-want-it-now, and they are linked to images of freedom and boundlessness. Showers are also associated with sport, with gyms and exercise, and with the toned, fit body that such pursuits support. They are also perceived to be 'cleaner' than baths, and thus chime in with modern preoccupations with the clean, pure, hygenisised body. Baths by contrast stress a different set of values. They are about relaxation, indulgence, luxury and retreat. At a simple level they represent a return to the womb: warm, wet and enclosing. They have the capacity to warm the whole body in a way that showers do not, something that commends them to people who live in cold and draughty houses. To that extent, showers in cold countries depend on a prior diffusion of central heating.

The rival discourses of showers and baths also reflect cultural imagery around masculinity and femininity. Kira, in his analysis of films and adverts, shows how these draw on the long historical association of bathing with luxury, extravagance and eroticism – the prerogatives of femininity in western culture (Kira 1967). Films often depicted beautiful and elegant women in their baths, and adverts for bath products draw on what Kira terms 'hetaeral or Pompadour' fantasies in which luxury and sensuality are linked. Men never feature in adverts for baths; they are only ever depicted showering. As we have seen the imagery of showers contains a number of masculine themes. Showers are vigorous, energetic, efficient, Spartan. Kira suggests that standing naked, buffeted by the water conveys a free and elemental condition that is attractive to urban American man. Showers are masculine when used by a man and neutral when by a women. Writing in the 1960s, Kira analyses shower adverts that do feature women in terms of the 'pal' image in which such women are seen as lively, modern and wholesome; and he makes a link to the way in which women in the period are moving into a man's world and acting symbolically like men. As we shall see, there are parallels here between his analysis and the rise of the slim, toned body for women with its androgynous ideal and rejection of overt or traditional female eroticism.

The ambivalences of the body in high modernity

High modernity – as opposed to postmodernity – conceptualises the modern world in terms of the intensification and radicalisation of processes of change already underway, and it does not represent the degree of cultural break that the term postmodernity implies. It is thus a more appropriate term to use in analysing changes in relation to the body and bathing, where, as we have seen, there has been a continuity of change over several centuries. Shilling (1993) has argued that in conditions of high modernity, the body assumes a new significance as a focus of personal identity and control. The earlier religious world view constructed and sustained ontological certainty outside the individual; but with secularisation, meaning has become fragmented and privatised (Berger 1973). People seek salvation through the rival regimes of the body. The body in the west has become a bearer of symbolic value, part of the project of self-identity, something to be worked upon, developed and refined. Where once the body was disciplined as part of religious practice in pursuit of spiritual goals, now the same techniques of fasting, denial and purification are used to support this-worldly goals of success, pleasure and consumption. These processes Turner (1984) terms 'secular asceticism'. He argues that body maintenance practices need to be seen as offering pseudo liberation through consumption. The body is disciplined so that it may consume more and better. This new hedonism is not oppositional in any way, but perfectly geared to the requirements of advanced capitalism.

In consumer culture there is a shift from the old production-oriented virtues of frugality to the new consumption-oriented values of expenditure and display. The body becomes something to be packaged, marketed and sold. An increasing emphasis is placed on its appearance and presentation. Williams and Bendelow (1998) express this in terms of the move from bodies producing commodities to commodities producing bodies. It is part of the particular dynamic of the body in consumer society that its ideals are unattainable. Advertising and the media present images of bodies and their perfection that cannot be achieved by ordinary people; and that is part of how they create the endless aspiration and its deflection into desire for the goods. In consumer culture our relationship with goods rests on their capacity not to satisfy needs but incite desires; and the project of the self becomes transformed into the possession of desired goods. More profoundly, such aspirations around the body are doomed to fail because the processes of aging and death cannot be held back. Consumer culture is youth oriented; and the perfect bodies it deals in are very young (photographic levels of perfection in models now require that they be in their teens). For Bauman (1992) the endless emphasis on resisting age that is characteristic of body maintenance movements and their extension in health education represents attempts, in the absence of any deeper cultural meaning, to defer the existential challenge of death.

The evaluation of the body in high modernity is hedged around with ambivalence. Much of the account of the body in the twentieth century rests on images of freedom, release, pleasure, desire, and this is constructed in particular against an image of Victorian past in which bodily life was shrouded, repressed, hidden and denied. One of the key images of modernism is sunshine, in which health-bringing light floods into the dark places and dark fears of the past, and light, easy clothes replace the dark, heavy constriction of the past. The image of the beach encapsulates this feeling, epitomising freedom, relaxation, playfulness, sexuality and ease. But the beach also has another, darker, side. It is a place of surveillance, where bodies are on view, monitored against standards that increasingly derive from the images promoted by the media and advertising, images that we have noted are unattainable. As a result the beach is also a place of anxiety and failure. The new body maintenance regimes are themselves far from joyful or body celebratory, but rest on punishing schedules of exercise, dieting and control.

These ambivalences of the body in high modernity can perhaps best be illustrated in relation to dieting and the ideal of slimness. The rise of the new slim ideal for women in the twentieth century and the related phenomena of eating disorders has been the subject of a large literature (Bordo 1993, MacSween 1993). It is a complex phenomena and I will refer here only to one of the themes that underlies it – ambivalence around femininity. The new body ideal manages to be both sexual and asexual at the same time. Being slim is perceived by individual women and wider culture as attractive and sexual; and the slim ideal is a sexy one. And yet, it is also androgynous and asexual, promoting an ideal of women's bodies that approaches the male form: slim hips, flat stomach, toned and slightly muscular body. Above all it is hatred and fear of 'fat' that informs the new ideology and lies at the core of its malign version in the form of eating disorders. This fear of flesh involves a denial and repression of traditional 'feminine' characteristics in the sense of flowing curves, billowing breasts, rounded hips and thighs. The new slimness is also about youthfulness; and the ideal it presents is that of a young girl not a mature woman. (Nancy Reagan in the 1980s epitomised this ideal of a woman in her sixties with the figure of a teenager.) Part of the meaning of the new slimness is a rejection of motherhood as woman's prime destiny, and its rise links historically to women's growing involvement in the labour market and in the masculine world of work. Women who work in male dominated areas of employment are required to repress the symbols of overt femininity or sexuality, while still not losing all identity as women. The new slim ideal assists in this, as well as acting as a general sign of control and discipline in life. Fatness is increasingly read as indulgence, failure and lack of control, and demonstrating control is central in the new body politics (and is carried forward in an exaggerated and pathological form in anorexia).

Modern attitudes to cleanliness contain something of the same ambivalences, promoting a body that is fresh, clean, wholesome, yet by the same token antiseptic, deodorised, sterile and asexual. In relation to smell, Corbin (1986) argues, we have seen a cultural retreat away from pleasure in strong body odours. The discrediting of musk as a basis for perfume and its replacement in the late eighteenth century by lighter, floral-based scents marks, he argues, a shift from the wish of women to emphasise the sexual and animal aspects of the body and its desires towards a wish to mask them; and such changes in the evaluation of smell parallel the rise of the new concern with cleanliness. By the end of the nineteenth century it was still possible to speak of *bouquet de corsage*, the attractive smell of perspiration in the ballroom. By the 1930s this had become BO.

Dirty dying and the unbounded body

We can now turn to see how this new perfectionism concerning the body has implications for the care sector. I discussed in Chapter 1 the relative paucity of gerontological work in this area in terms of a reluctance to engage with the 'negativity of the body'. One piece of work that does do so is Lawton's account of the processes of what she terms 'dirty dying', and in this she links what is happening in hospices with the developments in relation to the body in high modernity. Lawton (1998) starts from noting that as a result of active home care policies and pressure on through-put, few patients now die, or spend long periods, in the hospice, but that there is a subgroup that do. These are patients she terms 'unbounded', whose physical deterioration has reached such a state, particularly in relation to incontinence, rotting, disfigurement, that it has become impossible to maintain the boundaries of their bodies. Their care cannot be accommodated within the community either practically or symbolically. At this point, patients and carers, repelled by what was happening to the disintegrating body, often requested admission to the hospice. Smell was a particularly significant precipitator of this, and brought about a further marginalisation within the hospice. Patients, the smell of whose rotting tumours filled the air, presented serious problems for the hospice and its staff. Other patients often refused to speak to them, or to share a room, and relatives ceased to visit. They were often moved into side rooms. Hospices themselves gloss over these aspects of their work. Lawton's argument is that it is not death that is taboo in the hospice, but bodily disintegration and unboundedness. The effect of this on the patients was profound. They seemed to undergo a total loss of self, going through a radical process of withdrawal and disengagement. It was not that they attempted to transcend their decaying bodies so much as that their very selfhood was annihilated, leaving just the empty body behind. Some refused to speak even to close relatives, other refused to drink in the attempt to hasten death, others requested total sedation.

Lawton makes sense of this terrible account in terms of the growing intolerance in the West of the unbounded body. As a result certain sorts of bodily deterioration, demise and decay are set apart from mainstream society, and sequestered in the hospice. Hospices and other such institutions are there to: 'enable certain ideas about living, personhood and the hygienic, sanitised, somatically bounded body to be symbolically enforced and maintained.'(1998: 123) In the contemporary West, identity and selfhood are dependent upon the possession of a physically bounded body. In other cultures and societies identity is more a relational concept; personhood is less fixed and individual, more fluid and permeable. With this, Lawton argues, goes a different attitude to the body and its boundaries. In cultural contexts where people are not thought of as having a singular authentic identity mapped on to a singular separate body, substances emitted from the body are not seen as waste or dirt in quite the same way as they are in the contemporary western paradigm. This is why smell is particularly significant. It extends the patient's corporeality in ways that intrude and seep into other person's spaces. Odours by their nature cannot be easily contained; they escape and cross boundaries. This boundary transgressing quality acts 'to threaten the abstract and impersonal regime of modernity' (Classen *et al.* 1994: 5). It runs counter to our modern world view with its emphasis on discrete, defined divisions and on individual privacy. Smell and disintegration undermine current individualistic constructions of the person as stable, bounded and autonomous.

Conclusion

The purpose of this chapter has been to disturb our common sense understandings of what bathing is about, and to suggest some of the complexity that underlies what might otherwise seem a mundane and straightforward topic. Bathing has historically been located in a variety of discourses, of which the currently dominant discourse of hygiene is not the only, or even predominant, one. This has implications for how we understand the provision of bathing within community care, for the meanings of bathing are wider and more multiple than the traditional account of social policy would suggest. We need to widen our horizons and take in the variety and diversity of these meanings. For example, washing and bathing draw on perennial symbolism concerning water and the body; and we have seen the frequent connection with rituals of purification and rites of passage. These meanings contribute something to our understanding of baths in community care through their role in the day-to-day patterning of domestic life, as well as in settings such as prisons and hospitals. Baths have also been part of coercive cultures in which bodies are made subject to discipline, rendered docile through the application of technologies of dominance. Though bathing, as it takes place within community care, does not usually have these meanings, it contains distant echoes of them, in potentiality at least.

The meaning and symbolism of bathing is thus not fixed, but has been located in a range of discourses and connected with a variety of social practices. Elements that have at times been linked, can separate out, and come to have distinct and different meanings, as we saw in relation to the history of public baths, and the now diverse connotations of the word 'bath'. Elements that have been integral to bathing, can disappear or relocate to other social spaces. For example, one of the most striking changes in relation to bathing concerns the loss of the communal element that marks out the activity in the Roman, Japanese and medieval traditions. Baths were once primarily about conviviality; whereas today they are private activities, by and large performed alone. Indeed the new culture of bathing is one that emphasises individualism and privacy.

Bathing not only has its history, but its politics also, as we saw in relation to its links with Romanticist political theories concerning freedom and nature. Bathing in cold fresh water has in the past been associated with the rejection of *ancien régime* values, with their emphasis on superficial, vestimentary codes of cleanliness. In the nineteenth century this new bourgeois ethic underwrote growing social division in relation to the emergence of class society, as social distance became marked out in bodily habits, so that smell entered the history of class conflict. Economic and material developments have also played a part. The new culture of cleanliness rests on a diffusion of material affluence and the development of an industrial society capable of producing abundant hot water, soap and bathroom facilities. Initially in the nineteenth and early twentieth centuries this applied only to the middle classes, but in the post-war era, has been extended to society as a whole. The elaboration of bathroom goods, the multiplication of bathrooms and the intensification of bathing and washing are all products of late twentieth century affluence. But they also reflect wider social shifts, in particular growing individualism and separation in relation to the body. We saw how, contrary to some of our easy assumptions about the greater freedom accorded to bodily life in modern society, the story in relation to washing and bathing is one of new and more stringent demands being placed on the body. Under regimes of high modernity, the body assumes a new significance, and as part of this new levels of performance and control are demanded of it.

Community care is not isolated from such cultural trends. Being clean, not smelling, has become a necessary element in social inclusion, to the extent that the capacity to keep clean – as to have an adequate diet – has become a form of social right, something that few would be happy to deny to another, at least openly. The new emphasis on cleanliness also has implications for the experience of the body in old age, and for forms of disability like incontinence that challenge that perfectionism.

We need thus to conceptualise community care within a wider context of meanings that has traditionally been the case. Exploring the historical significance of bathing and washing enables us to do this, questioning current approaches to service delivery and analysis that rest on too limited an understanding of social life and its meanings; and in doing so it contributes to the wider project of what Lewis (2000) has termed 'expanding the social policy imaginary'.

3   Bathing, washing and the management of personal care

Help with bathing and washing involves nakedness, touch and the transgression of the normal boundaries of adult life. To receive such help thus represents one of the great watersheds of aging or disability. In the chapter that follows I will explore what this involved for individuals in the study (mainly older people, but including some younger physically disabled: the study is described more fully in the Appendix), looking at the meanings they ascribed to bathing and showering, their feelings about their bodies, and their preferences in regard to the sources of such care. Bathing, like all personal care, contains transgressive aspects and the chapter will explore how these are negotiated and their significance for the ambivalent forms of closeness that are created by such care.

Personal care

Bathing and washing need to be seen in the wider context of personal care. 'Personal care' is defined in terms of those things that an adult would normally do for him or herself; it marks the point at which 'self-servicing' becomes the norm (though of course that point of self servicing has shifted historically). You may have meals made for you, clothes ironed and laid out, domestic life smoothed by wives or servants, but even the richest bath themselves and wipe their own bottoms. Only the very young or people who cannot manage are helped in these ways; and this is a powerful source of the infantalising tendency in carework. This social symbolism is difficult to resist; it is hard to maintain adulthood or dignity in the face of being fed with a spoon, having your pads changed or your face and body washed. The loss of bodily control whether over limbs or bowels threaten the return to a pre-adult status. We have already noted the particular difficulties that incontinence and other forms of bodily unboundedness pose for modern sensibility with its emphasis on the 'purified' body, contained, individual and clearly bounded. Personal care breaches those boundaries; and it involves negotiating the intimacies of touch and nakedness.

Nakedness

Culture provides us with almost no images of the aging body unclothed, so that when we do encounter the reality of such, it comes as a visual shock. Partly this is a result of the representational tradition of the west, dominated by the Classical and Renaissance depiction of the nude, in which the body is presented in idealised form and in which its beauty and perfection are expressions of aesthetic and moral ideals (Clark 1956). Media images of the old are notably sparse. Adverts rarely depict older people, and there is an almost total ban on the depiction of older bodies. The dominance of these images means that we experience divergence from the ideal in terms of decline, decay and failure. We have little sense culturally of aesthetic pleasure in old flesh, or of what a beautiful old body might look like. Shifts in culture associated with the new, postmodern pre-occupation with the body and its perfection reinforce such judgements. Older people thus experience their aging bodies in the context of a profound cultural silence.

The social meaning of nakedness is closely associated with intimacy, and in modern western culture particularly with sexual intimacy. The link between nakedness and closeness is both a direct one, in that nakedness permits actual physical touch and closeness; and a metaphorical one, in that to be naked is to divest oneself of protection and disguise. Clothes are central in the public presentation of self; they disguise our bodies and bring them more into accord with the social ideal; and they express our social position and individual personality. To be without them is to be without these supports. Nakedness thus creates vulnerability, as well as intimacy. Within erotic relationships, we experience the process of undressing in a dual way. Uncovering the body below the clothes is paralleled by uncovering the person below the social persona. Literal undressing and emotional undressing operate in parallel. But this process really only applies in the modern west to erotic relations. Though with friends, as we get to know them better, there is a growth of intimacy and trust so that one begins to get below the social exterior, but there is no parallel physical process. There may be some loosening up of bodily presentation as people get to be more at ease with one another, but there is no literal uncovering, so that for these relations the naked self remains only a metaphor. This is in contrast to erotic relationships where the metaphor and the direct experience are mutually reinforcing. The strength of this experience means that to be naked in a social context always has some erotic element in it. This has implications for the bathing encounter and for the kinds of intimacy that it creates. Nakedness here strikes a discordant note that disturbs normal social reality. To be naked in a social and not erotic context is odd and disjunctive and it has therefore to be presented in terms of a bounded form of intimacy from which the sexual has been consciously excluded.

The charged nature of the encounter is also affected by the fact that the nakedness is asymmetrical. The older or disabled person is naked, but the worker is not, and this creates a considerable discrepancy of power. The fact of this is widely understood, and underlies such practices as denying prisoners or patients their clothes, or of interrogating suspects naked – processes designed to demean the individual and create vulnerability and compliance; and it is in order to reduce such effects that doctors and nurses are taught to examine patients in such a way as to limit their bodily exposure (Wolf 1988, Lawler 1991).

Touch

Touch has profound emotional significance. Preceding speech as a form of communication, it takes us back to our earliest experiences. Tactile metaphors are about feelings, emotions, relations with others. Skin is the largest sense organ of the body, and the major part of our experience of embodiment derives from tactility (Montagu 1986, Synnott 1993). In general the literature on touch has concluded that modern western society is less tactile compared with non-western societies and the historical past. The decline of touch is be linked to debates about modernity in which the growing impersonality of modern life is reflected in a retreat from bodily contact, reflecting the general trend towards greater individuation and separation in the management of the body explored in Chapter 2 in relation to smell and personal cleanliness. Victorian photographs do seem to show more in the way of casual arm touching and body leaning in the past, certainly between individuals of the same sex. Montagu (1986) argues that touch in modern life has become increasingly confined to erotic relations, so that adults, particularly men, live in a world that is largely atactile except for sex. This is particularly damaging, he argues, for older people left without the comfort of regular touch.

Touch in relation to the body is structured according to gradations of intimacy and power (Jourard 1966, Jourard and Rubin 1968). Different parts of the body may be touched by different people according to gender and the closeness of the relationship. Touch is also a vector of status, authority and dominance, with the more powerful touching the less powerful, superiors touching inferiors (Henley 1973). There is a gendered pattern to this, with women more likely to be touched than men. Henley interprets this in terms of their subordinate position within patriarchy; though it may also reflect the greater tactility of women's lives; women remaining to some extent more embedded in a traditional world of connectedness. There is also evidence that while women evaluate touch by a service provider in a positive way, men do not, associating it with the inferiority and dependence that they have been socialised to reject (Whitcher and Fischer 1979). Men are also more likely to regard touch in a sexualised way, interpreting male touch in terms of homosexuality (Sussman and Rosenfeld 1978, Whitcher and Fisher 1979, Routasalo and Isola 1996).

Accepting personal care

The changes imposed by the loss of function in old age are massive. When people speak of the rigidity of people in old age or their reluctance to accept change, they fail to grasp the magnitude of this. Most people in the sample dealt with such change in a stoical way. Raging against its realities was seen as a route to pain and unhappiness, and the dominant approach was one of acceptance and of taking each day as it came. It was partly for this reason that it was often difficult to get elderly people to expand on how they managed bathing before, or what they missed about it now. Going down that route for them was unproductive and a reminder of what they had lost; and respondents were resistant to questions that tried to get them to explore these areas. Facing forward, keeping positive and taking things as they came was the dominant approach.

Baths and bathing

Attitudes to bathing now and in the past varied among the respondents. For some, baths had always been a luxury and source of pleasure. Mrs Kennelly whose severe Parkinson's meant that she could no longer have a bath, looked back with nostalgia on the experience: 'I'd love to be able to get in the bath. Just lay there and splash it over ... wallow in it. Lovely.' Sir Peter, a former naval officer, had been in the habit of bathing twice a day, an enthusiasm he attributed to years of deprivation in the cramped conditions of warships. Mr Wagstaffe, who had been the manager of a private dining club, also enjoyed baths, though he drew the line at their elaboration:

> Well I've always liked baths ... I have some friends who have cups of tea or drinks or things in the bath. I've never fancied it. It's like breakfast in bed, which is a thing I abhor. You finish up all bums and crumbs, don't you. It's not for me. But a straightforward bath yes.

Despite the dominant gendered imagery described in the last chapter, men as much as women expressed pleasure in bathing, underlining the disjunction between the representation of gender and the actual pattern of activity.

The coming of disability and the possibility that they would no longer be able to have a bath was for some a source of real distress. Mrs Fitzgerald, the widow of a successful surgeon, had always loved bathing:

> All my life, up in a morning, throw open the bed, into the bathroom – that's the way I lived. ... It's always been terribly important to me. And that's when I got panic-stricken when I thought I wasn't going to be able to have any bath.

For her the bathing service had come as a godsend: ' Though it's only once a week ... it's become the rose of my week, because though I'm used to bathing every day, it's such a joy.'

For these people, baths were not just about getting clean, but a source of pleasure and enjoyment in a wider sense. They could ease the aches and pains of the body. As Mrs Smythe explained: 'a hot bath.... I find it very comforting.' For some it was still a luxurious process even if they had to be helped. Mrs Napier explained how:

> We have nice foamy shower gel ... it's lovely like being a baby again. [Laughter] We have the flannel and I get the foamiest ... at the moment I'm using Johnsons Ph5 which is not very expensive but lovely and foamy.

For others, however, baths had never been that important. Many had not been frequent bathers, preferring to wash down with a flannel. For some, baths had always been matter-of-fact affairs, simply a means of getting clean; and they found it difficult to expand on the subject in the interview. They felt there was nothing much to say, and were puzzled by the subject of the research (in fact, all respondents were puzzled that a topic like bathing should be the subject of research).

Provision of help varied between the two study areas. In inner London, respondents either got help from a dedicated bathing service run by a voluntary sector organisation, or from the local authority home care service, or from private agencies. In the second study area, Coastville, there was no bathing service as such and people received help from a variety of public and private sector home care agencies as part of a package of personal care. The frequency of provision also varied. The voluntary sector bathing service in London only came once a week. A few respondents felt that was not enough. As Mr Wagstaffe said: 'I don't particularly want to have people open all the doors and windows when I go in anywhere. ... I don't think that once a week is a sufficient standard of cleanliness.' He paid privately to have someone come in addition. Between the weekly visits, Mrs Fitzgerald struggled on her own, trying to get clean by precarious means, balancing a basin on the toilet: 'I put a special thing on the seat ... the basin's there and the bath's there and I use many flannels and many towels. It's a proper mess – you can't imagine.' By and large, however, people were pleased with what they got, reflecting the general pattern of gratitude and low expectations found in most studies of older people. Some clients of home care did receive more frequent help, but this was not as part of a bathing service so much as what was termed a 'personal hygiene' package.

A 'proper bath'

Although this study – and the wider policy world – refers to 'baths' and 'bathing', for many people the help they received fell well short of what could be termed a proper bath. The concept of a 'proper bath' was recognised by everyone, recipients and providers alike: what it meant was getting down under the water, ideally with the freedom to move your legs, and to lean back. The problem was that enabling people to do this involved physical lifting, and this is increasingly forbidden under directives from the European Union relating to manual handling, enshrined in UK legislation on health and safety at work, which limit the weight that may be lifted by employees without mechanical assistance (Health and Safety Executive 1992). The concern is to prevent back injury, a common problem faced by care staff, and it means that staff cannot lift clients unaided, even when they are very light or frail, and they must use a hoist or other equipment. Few clients in fact have such equipment, and the cramped arrangements of many bathrooms and the side panel of the bath make using such things as a hoist, or manoeuvring the person down into the bath, awkward. As a result the majority of people in the study receiving a 'bath' did not receive a proper bath and were not able to get fully into the water. This limited the nature of the experience severely. As Mrs Bridgeman commented: 'I *long* to get my bum in the water (both laugh). It would be bliss you know.'

A small number of respondents were sufficiently mobile in their hips, and had enough strength in their arms and legs to get in and out with minor assistance. One or two only really needed help to balance, or the reassurance of knowing that someone was within call. Most however did not get a proper bath. They either sat on a board across the bath or on a small seat; and after having been helped to wash, had warm water poured over them. Though the careworkers acknowledged this was not as nice as a proper bath, they believed it was still a soothing and enjoyable experience. Crystal, a young careworker from the voluntary sector bathing scheme, explained how she spent a lot of time:

> Just pouring more and more water on their backs ... Water is very very relaxing and it just feels nice, it's a nice sensation to have warm water running on you ... also you feel a lot cleaner and fresher if you've had actual water pouring over you rather than just a cloth going like that ... I think it's just a nice physical sensation, relaxing and just you feel good about yourself, feel better in yourself.

However nice this experience, it was not a full bath. Only the full depth of water allows the person to experience the fluidity and warmth of the water, its buoyancy and freedom – factors that are particularly important when limbs are heavy or painful to move. By and large, respondents were resigned to this and grateful for what they got, but conflicts did sometimes arise. Some clients had had to be warned that if they attempted to pre-empt the situation by sitting down fully in the bath, the careworker would not help them get up, but simply ring for an ambulance. The potential humiliation was sufficient to keep most people in line.

Showers

From a managerial point of view, showers offer a practical solution to many of these problems. Clients can walk or be pushed in a chair into them; and the quick efficiency of their action means that the work can be accomplished speedily, and, as it were, dirty old bodies turned into clean ones. This was not how respondents saw it; and showers were almost universally rejected in the interviews. This was partly because most people in the study were not of a generation accustomed to their use, and few had experienced anything better than the ineffective gravity type. One or two clients who had been brought up abroad preferred a shower, but as the bathing manager commented: 'there is something quite English about soaking in a bath.'

Showers did not perform the same functions as baths. They did not warm the whole body in the ways that a hot bath could, something that is important in the context of the poor housing that many older people occupy. As Mr Wagstaffe explained: 'It's like coming out of the sea isn't it, freezing when you come out and the water dries on you. I think that's known as the release of latent heat, is it not?'

The discourse of showers is also, as we have seen, one of energy, youth, time saving and vigour. For many older people this imagery is disjunctive. Showers also leave less time for relaxing or talking. As Roz, a careworker in Coastville, explained:

> It's a more hurried experience than having a bath. ... If I was going in to bath somebody, and I would sort of like say, I'll run the bath now, and I could still talk to them while the bath was running, and then you know, say the bath's ready and ... then take them to the bathroom. With a shower it's sort of like you take them straight into where they're going to be showered, it's more of an initial shock, and quicker as well.

As the final sentence of the quotation shows, showers can also contain a sense of something that is done to you: the person is taken in and showered, and there is an 'initial shock'. In the subtle power dynamics of care there is a constant tension between taking a bath and being bathed in which the experience of showers reinforces the second.

Showers can also be a source of more practical anxieties. Respondents were worried about slipping, and standing under the water could be difficult. For some, the actual experience of the water raining down on their heads was unpleasant, even threatening one. Mrs Bucknell, the widow of a builder who had formally been in service explained: 'I don't like the water coming down over me all the time.' Some people found that being in a cabinet with the water pounding down was claustrophobic. Paul Hubbard, a young physically disabled man with cerebral palsy explained: 'The trouble with a shower is ... you're too enclosed and [you] can get too hot as well.' On occasions he had been scalded.

For many older women getting their hair wet was an added disadvantage. As women get older their hair becomes thinner and more difficult to manage, and this is one of the reasons why many older women, even of modest means, go regularly to the hairdresser. Showers disorder hair completely, and make it hard to reassemble the public persona. The head and face are always important in the presentation of self, but become all the more so once the body is frail and mobility lost. For some older men, washing the hair was anyway an alien procedure, accustomed as they were to frequent visits to the barber and very short hair. Desiree, a London careworker, complained about a client who refused to have his hair washed and who retorted when she tried:

'How dare you! I've never washed my hair in thirty-odd years.' I could not believe him. I went downstairs and I said to his wife 'I've just tried to get your husband to wash his hair and he's told me he hasn't washed it in thirty-odd years, could you confirm that?' She said 'Yeah' – she's been with him for that long and he's never washed his hair .... But he has someone in that sprays it and cuts it.

Embarrassment

Receiving help with bathing is a potentially embarrassing business. Most people in the study felt this to some degree, though many had became accustomed to the experience, or at least had learnt to accepted it as a matter of 'Hobson's choice', the term used by Mrs Elster. She was determined to stay living at home though she was confined to living on the bed. As she explained:

MRS ELSTER: Well at the beginning I didn't like being personally washed of course but after six years I haven't got any more hold ups about that, you know you just get on with it, get clean is my main thing ...

INTERVIEWER: Right so you get used to it or you just have to learn to put up with it?

MRS ELSTER: Well pretty well learn to put up with it, and really you do put up with a helluva lot.

Mrs Ostrovski, who was Polish, hated the whole experience much more deeply, but she had learnt to grit her teeth and survive by distancing herself psychologically: 'you pretend it doesn't matter', though for anyone who is not a 'cabbage' it is horrible to be helped 'in these intimate places ... There are some people who are very liberated and I don't know, they sunbathe and wash naked ... well I am too old, a generation not thinking that way.' Mrs Colegate had at first found that it was:

> an ordeal to have a bath originally, with people coming in, I must admit ... When you've been able to do it yourself for all those years, and then you've gotta rely on other people to do it, it takes some getting used to but ... now, doesn't worry me so much ... Now I look forward to em coming.

The careworkers concurred. Hazel, the manager of the voluntary sector bathing scheme, explained:

> A lot of them haven't even had their husband see them without clothes, so when any of us go in, it's like perhaps the first time and ... it's quite a big thing really, but after the first, second, third time, it's amazing, they're sort of coming from bedroom to bathroom with no clothes on, and you know they just lose all their inhibitions.

This sense of ease could however be fragile, and it often depended on familiarity with a particular worker. As Mrs Bucknell explained:

> I keep to Doreen, cos I'm happy with her because I'm really conscious of anybody seeing me ... I don't like the girls [other careworkers] seeing me undressed, er naked. Getting in the bath or anything like that.... I don't know why – but I just don't like it. And with Doreen, now, I was very nervous with her at first, but now I'm so accustomed that I take no notice.

A number of respondents would avoid having a bath if a substitute worker was sent. For these reasons frequent changes of staff were experienced as distressing. With each new person the whole process of taking your clothes off both metaphorically and literally had to be gone through yet again.

Some clients tried to manage their embarrassment by keeping some of their clothes on, though this could end up making the experience worse:

> He used to keep his shorts on you know and you know, I said by all means if that's what you want to do, but when it came to drying, and the whole thing was worse for him really, because when the shorts got wet, they stuck to him, so it was more bother getting them off. It was more embarrassing for him.

Another lady liked to keep her slip on, or at least did so with workers that she did not know. Miss Henderson similarly made a clear distinction between workers she knew, whom she was happy to have with her in the bathroom, and those who were strangers whom she preferred to remain out in the hall.

For many older people hospital was a major transition in their experience of their bodies. As Mr Wagstaffe commented: 'once you've been in hospital for a while, all ideas of privacy disappear straight down the drain, don't they.' Operations and investigations had stripped people of any remaining sense of modesty, though this indifference often seemed to be more a matter of alienation from the body rather than real ease. Mrs Ostrovski recounted the process as one of becoming an object, in which the only way to survive was to distance oneself:

> When you go to hospital, teaching hospital, and you are there and you have twenty students. You lie naked and the professor – you are becoming example of the things, and twenty people touch you, and you just close your mind, and you say yourself, *it doesn't matter, it doesn't matter, it doesn't matter* … You are really a subject. You are not a person.

Embarrassment is by its nature interactive. The cues that the other person gives can be as important in creating or dispelling embarrassment as feelings within the individual. Mrs Napier felt that the bathing aides were very good: 'I think the thing is that they're at ease themselves.' Kathryn, a careworker in Coastville explained how it was vital to convey the sense of really wanting to give someone a bath in a positive way in order to get over their inhibitions.

From the clients' point of view nothing was more horrible than the experience of being helped by someone who was repelled by the work. Mrs Ostrovski felt this with one careworker who was a trainee journalist and had been doing the work as a fill-in, though it was clear that she hated it:

> She thought it was absolutely disgusting to have anything to do with anything, but she had no option because there was no other – she wanted to be a newspaper woman. For a newspaper woman to wash somebody's behind, it's too far a stretch. So you felt you know, you felt she is doing you such a favour, you prefer not to – you prefer to stink actually.

The fact that the careworkers were accustomed to doing the work, and were by and large at ease with it, did not always resolve the issue of embarrassment. As Sharon Kimpton explained what mattered to her was not *their* ease, but how *she* felt:

> I know like they all say: 'Oh, I've seen one body, I've seen them all.' But they haven't seen *mine* – it doesn't matter how many times they say: 'Oh I've seen loads of people, I've seen loads of people having a bath, I've helped loads of people have a bath', but not *me*, you know, and it doesn't make you feel any better them saying that.

She linked this sense of embarrassment directly to her age (she was in her thirties) and to her sense of herself as a potentially sexually active woman: 'this is embarrassing ... because I'm not a child any more, because I'm a woman, because I've got all my bits, you know.'

Doing the work was itself no guarantee that the worker would feel all right about receiving such help should they have to. Roz, a careworker in Coastville, was adamant that she would hate to be bathed; she could not contemplate or tolerate the prospect.

ROZ: If you came into this room now and said to me I was gonna bath you, I couldn't, I'd say no, I'd rather not have a bath, didn't make any difference to me you know, whether I was filthy or whatever, or I felt really uncomfortable I would still say no, I don't want a bath, thank you very much.

INTERVIEWER: Why would you say that, do you think?

ROZ: Because to me that's private, to me I want to wash myself, I
don't want somebody else to wash me and I don't, I certainly
don't want somebody else to dry me and put my clothes on to
me afterwards ... I'd rather be smelly and I'm absolutely sure.

It is important to emphasise that not all clients were embarrassed:
'Most of them aren't shy at all, they just come in and take their
clothes off and walk around they don't really mind,' Sophie who
worked for the London bathing scheme commented. Mrs Napier said
that she was never embarrassed in front of the careworker: 'Oh
gracious no, I've walked round in my birthday suit without any
trouble at all.' Some older people were quite uninhibited. Stella
recounted the antics of one old lady keen to show how life still
coursed though her veins:

> Just stands up in the bath and goes like this you know does a
> little dance ....The whole thing is kind of a pursuit in proving
> how agile and full of life she is, and I mean I do love that, see
> that to me is very energising, I just go in to an environment
> where somebody's just so full of life you know. And she's sup-
> posedly at the end of her life you know, the last bits of her life,
> and she's not. It's that kind of love of just being in that little
> wicked body of hers, and doing a dance with a towel right in the
> middle of the bath.

For some respondents the sense of not being embarrassed appeared
to have a class dimension. Miss Garfield when asked if she liked to
have a regular person replied in an upper-class drawl: 'From the
bathing point of view, I don't give a damn.... it doesn't worry me in
the slightest.' When asked about people being modest, she replied
'I'm afraid I'm not modest at all, you know. Why a grown person
should be modest I don't know.' Mrs Smythe, another upper-middle-
class woman was similar surprised by people who were embarrassed
about such things: 'So I don't think I am easily embarrassed, no. ... I
think people are sometimes rather – over-modest, I call it.'

Parts of the body

Different parts of the body were managed and treated differently by
both clients and careworkers. In general this followed the pattern
familiar from the literature on touch in which contact with the body
is structured in terms of intimacy and closeness (Jourard 1966,

Jourard and Rubin 1968). In general, upper arms and back are relatively neutral and may be touched by most people; knees and thighs less so; and breasts and genitals are off limits in all but erotic relations. Most clients preferred to wash their genital and anal area themselves. As Mrs Bridgeman, who had worked as a secretary in the Australian embassy, explained: 'The Australians have a saying: "A P C": armpits and crotches. (Both laugh). So that's what you have to do, you know. And as I say I can manage the top of me and, and my crotches.' Mrs Bucknell, who had been in service, was clear that she liked to manage for herself: 'I always wash underneath myself – I won't let her do it .... She would do underneath if I let her, but I said "No, if you don't mind Doreen I'd rather do it myself." '

Clients often expressed relief that at least they were spared what they saw as the indignity of being washed in these more intimate parts; and careworkers were sometimes reluctant to get involved with intimate contact. Mrs Elster, who did need this sort of help, remarked on:

> one girl who doesn't like to wash you below, and so she doesn't dare, but if you say, 'Oh will you just do a little bit more there.' Oh! Private. I think she thinks it's sexual or something, maybe. I can't understand cos she's youngish, twenty-three I think.

In her interview the careworker explained that she was indeed squeamish:

ZARA: I think I'd prefer to wash a man fully than to wash a woman fully. Because I do get a bit squeamish when it comes to dealing with ladies private parts. I don't mind if it's the bottom, the top half, but then once it comes to, you know, cos I've always been brought up to know that that part you deal with yourself or someone that is close to you, deals with that area. But men, I think I'd wash him anyhow, you know just wash them, if it's a man, cos I know that, you know, it is the opposite sex kind of thing. It does sound a bit funny but, that's just me.

INTERVIEWER: So you feel, you feel easier in a way dealing with a man's private parts?

ZARA: Well, not exactly his private parts, but when it comes to washing men, you know, I'll just wash them down and stuff. A woman I would wash her down as well, but once it come to like, inserting and to like creaming round that area I am, you know a bit, squeamish to that.

Careworkers often rationalised their reluctance by saying that nearly all clients could manage that much of their care and it was good to encourage independence.

The bottom was regarded as slightly less sensitive than the genitals: 'I don't think that's so sort of worrying', remarked one careworker. Attempts by male clients to get careworkers to touch their private parts were not uncommon, and we shall see in Chapter 7 how this was dealt with along with other sexual advances.

One part of the body was repeatedly emphasised by both clients and careworkers: the back. In the interviews the back was deployed metonymically to designate the whole body, and washing the back repeatedly stood for the process of bathing itself. For many respondents this presented a more acceptable way of talking about an otherwise intimate process. In the hierarchy of touch, the back is not a sensitive area; it is somewhere, in conjunction with the upper arm, that can be touched in a relatively open way by most people. Touching the back, giving it a vigorous unrestrained wash was something reported with pleasure by clients and careworkers; 'they do enjoy it, that you know, a lot of people really, "Oooh", you know, "give my back a good rub." ' Asking for contact in this area appeared acceptable. The back is also, in the nature of the bath encounter, the part of the body that faces the careworker and that shelters and hides more vulnerable and private parts. Putting an arm across the back, around the body is a relatively neutral way for the careworker to make human contact. So the back comes to stand for the body and for the person, providing an opportunity for an intimacy and closeness that still retains a certain neutrality about it.

Old bodies and nice standards

A number of older people in the sample had internalised a sense of their bodies as no longer pleasant, and as something that might be distasteful to have to manage. Mrs Fitzgerald explained: 'They're so young and beautiful, it must be awful for them to have to handle old, awkward bodies.' Sir Peter felt: 'It's rather bad luck on the girls, scrubbing old gentlemen's backs.' Mrs Fitzgerald added: 'They're wonderful people. ... I must say, I mean they must have something inside them because – it's not the sort of thing – I don't know when I was young whether I would have wanted to have looked after old people.' Mrs Kennelly felt the same: 'I say to them, "I feel sorry for you, getting up in the morning and this is the kind of job you've got to do", you know, not very nice.' Later she explained how she felt 'dreadful' about having to ask a young girl to help her. 'This young girl, … twenty eight, beautiful girl. She's very pretty, and there's the ugly lump. Oh dear!'

It was clear that some of the response related to the age of the worker. When asked directly, most recipients said that age did not matter to them; the character of the careworker was more important, and some indeed enjoyed young people coming to the house. But a number did make a qualification about very young careworkers, which for them meant those in their twenties or younger. Partly these young workers were perceived as flighty and ignorant of housework, but there was also an issue about the body. Many older recipients seemed to feel more at ease with workers whose bodies were themselves no longer in a perfect state of youth.

A number of female respondents consciously presented themselves in terms of nice standards, of fastidiousness in relation to their bodies and keeping clean. They emphasised how they kept different flannels for above and below, and were careful to maintain standards of hygiene. This was not a result of probing in the interview, but something they spontaneously raised. In part these appeared to be statements about themselves in the past and of continuity with that old self. But it also seemed part of keeping age at bay, an assertion of status against the fear of decline, a repudiation of the category of the old and smelly. What underlies this is the strength of the negative perceptions of the old in culture, perceptions that older people have to a considerable degree themselves internalised.

The response was a gendered one. No men in the study made a point of emphasising their high standards. Women are socialised to be more fastidious in relation to their bodies, something that was seen as part of femininity. Men, by contrast, are not encouraged or required to internalise ideals of niceness of standards – indeed they are allowed to be slightly messier and smellier as part of a rough masculinity (Classen *et al.* 1994). To be overly concerned with cleaning or deodorising the body is regarded as slightly effeminate. Men also may be able to get away with lower standards of hygiene as part of a generalised feeling of being at home in the world – of not having to fit in – compared to women. Obelkevich (1994), however, suggests that social shifts resulting in greater power for women have produced pressures on men to improve their standards of hygiene. The gendered response also draws on a wider social mysogynies concerning women's bodies, particularly their genitals (Greer 1986, Ardener 1987). Women's genitals are presented in patriarchal discourse with deep ambivalence, sources of both desire and revulsion, and women internalise this ambivalence in terms of anxieties around their bodies and their acceptability. Mrs Colegate explained obliquely:

MRS COLEGATE: I think ladies need a soak occasionally.
INTERVIEWER: Why do you?
MRS COLEGATE: Well I don't know, I think you know, its nice.
INTERVIEWER: Sort of psychologically need a soak, or to get properly clean or ...?
MRS COLEGATE: Well perhaps to get properly clean, mmm.

Help with bathing involves direct touch. It was hard to get clients to talk openly about this in the interviews. It was too intimate a territory for easy exploration. The sexualised character of touch in the west makes it difficult to acknowledge social pleasure in touch. Respondents shied away from the idea that bathing might involve touch that itself brought pleasure or comfort. Touch is also a form of communication that lies below words, and expressing its significance in words can seem awkward and disjunctive. For some older people the inhibition also related to the sense that touching them was not an enjoyable thing for the careworker to have to do. As we have seen some older people in the sample had internalised a 'truth' about the unpleasing nature of their bodies. Mrs Ostrovski was conscious that some people did not like to touch the bodies of old people.

There are people who old body make uneasy. They have sort of thing about touching.... It's in the air. Nobody would *dare* to say anything to you, but you can feel the (pause) – you feel it. It's not a ... nobody can control the other person who feels like that. Cannot control either, however hard. Because these things are subconscious, likes or dislikes, so I mean, you wouldn't like to touch the snake.

Her perception is supported by other evidence that shows that nurses are less likely to touch older patients (Montagu 1986). Mrs Ostrovski felt that staff often forced themselves, but that the basic dislike remained.

MRS OSTROVSKI: Quite a lot of people, even doctors, you can *feel* (pauses) conscience will (pauses) – Somebody touches you but you feel he touches you because he's supposed to touch you. You know what I mean.

INTERVIEWER: So they know they're meant to touch?
MRS OSTROVSKI: Yes.
INTERVIEWER: But you don't feel they really want to?
MRS OSTROVSKI: You feel there is – they *must* touch, but they
   don't touch. It's some sort of a *conscious* touching.

She added: 'I would prefer to have nobody than to have somebody
who would be sick each time they're supposed to touch me.'
   The careworkers found it easier to discuss the role of touch in
their work, but even here there was a certain reluctance to regard it
as openly part of the service. As with the clients, this seemed to imply
straying into ambiguous territory, and they preferred to separate
intimate touch from social closeness. The exception to this was
Stella, a New Age influenced careworker, who was unusual in her
open articulation of the role of touch in her work. She saw it as
something that lay below and beyond the level of words; and she
enjoyed the deeper intimacy that this hands-on work brought. She
explained how she was someone who needed to get in deep and close
with people, but that the nature of modern society did not often
allow this. Carework gave her that:

> And you're only latch into that with people you know once in a
> while [that deeper closeness] whereas you get that every day and
> call it work (both laugh). It's really nice, it's like keeps you going
> ... I personally have a sort of a high intensity need and it really
> fills that for me, like I, it's often hard for me to get in deep
> enough for to you know, and that's not where people are at most
> of the time.

The majority of careworkers, however, did not see touch in bathing
work as a route to greater closeness, and some indeed saw it as a
barrier. As Roz commented: 'It's a bit more *personal* [said with a
negative emphasis] than giving somebody a cuddle.' They were warm
and tactile in their responses, but they preferred to emphasise the
social touch of cuddles and kisses, rather than intimate bathing help
as a route to emotional closeness.
   This was in contrast to nurses. Nursing literature, particularly in
its holistic variants, is full of praise for the role of touch in nursing
practice; indeed it has become something of a watchword in the
assertion of nursing values as against managerialist and technocratic
erosion (van der Riet 1997). The community nurses in the study were
happy to endorse the role of touch:

It's the most intimate thing you will ever do for someone. [It is] very special to nursing ... a bond you get with someone, maybe just ... from being tactile with each other, certainly that you wouldn't ever get in a very intimate partner relationship. So maybe that's what you enjoy, is sort of being tactile with people. That's a typical nursing trait isn't it being quite tactile.

It seemed that their professional status, together with the wider ideology of holistic medical practice, meant that touch could be openly acknowledged, in contrast to the less developed ideology of carework, where the potentially transgressive aspects of touch were not contained within professional boundaries.

Cross-gender tending: an asymmetrical relationship

There is an asymmetry in the treatment of men's and women's bodies in culture that has implications for the care encounter. This applies both to the bodies of clients and to gendered assumptions about who may have access to them. There are three key elements in the construction of this asymmetry. The first concerns assumptions about sexuality, largely male sexuality; the second, the link between women and motherhood, and by extension women and all forms of intimate tending; and the third, the treatment of men and women's bodies in wider culture, in particular the imposition of modesty and conceal-ment on women's bodies. I will discuss the first two in greater detail in Chapter 6 which discusses male careworkers, and Chapter 7 which explores the construction of carework. Here we will simply note that these assumptions are also significant in relation to clients' feelings about cross-gender tending.

Women's bodies have traditionally been prime sites of control within patriarchy. One of the main forms this takes is the imposition of rules of modesty, whereby women's bodies are more hidden and controlled than those of men. The most vivid example is the use of purdah and the veil within Muslim culture. Though located in a particular and very different tradition from that of the west, it illustrates a common pattern whereby codes of modesty and corporeal seclusion for one sex are used to control sexuality generally. Women are here confined to the private sphere; thus creating a free, public arena in which men can act unencumbered – theoretically at least – by the complexities of sexuality, emotion and intimate life. Women experience the imposition of such rules in a dual way, both as a concealment of what is coveted, and as a threat of shame and embarrassment; and modesty is the internalisation of this duality.

In relation to washing and bathing, there are a number of examples of this asymmetrical pattern of modesty and concealment. In the nineteenth century boys and men traditionally swam naked in the rivers, whereas such behaviour was not possible for women (indeed they were forced to avert their gaze) (Raverat 1952). Once women did become involved in public swimming, costumes were required for both sexes. Similarly public urinals permit men to urinate in a more open way that is allowed to women (even after questions of clothing and relative exposure are taken into account); and indeed the lack of access to such facilities in the nineteenth century was a factor limiting the freedom of women to move about the public space of the city. This pattern of male freedom and female seclusion is echoed today in the changing areas of public baths, where it is common for the male side to be collective, but the female to have cubicles. In certain milieus, the demands of modesty have been so totalising that they apply even to the female self when alone: in convent schools it used to be customary for girls to wear a shift even when bathing alone (Goubert 1989). It is worth noting how at a symbolic representational level, nakedness and exposure and men's and women's bodies are treated rather differently. There has been a relatively high cultural toleration since the Renaissance (legitimated by the prestige of classical culture) of female nudity in the idealised form of public statuary and images. This is less so in relation to men, or at least the genitals of men, so that public exposure is more circumscribed.

Women's bodies are also more protected in the sense that they are often presented as requiring more in the way of care and caution. Men are expected to take a rougher, more robust attitude to their physicality. Boys are socialised to be daring and vigorous, particularly through the medium of sport; girls to be more cautious and controlled. Girls are encouraged to deploy their bodies more tentatively, in ways that protect and hide (Young 1990, Connell 1995).

Women's bodies are thus more shrouded and covered up, hidden from a male phallic gaze. The rules of modesty apply primarily to women, and there are not the same demands in relation to men. Women's bodies are more confined within the private sphere; access is traditionally limited. Women are hidden or exposed, and access to them by men is gained or granted. Access to the bodies of men does not operate for women in the same way. This links to traditional conservative discourses of sexuality wherein women are passive, the objects of desire in men, and allow men to have sex with them (or withhold permission) but do not seek it for themselves. Women in this account use sex to achieve other things – a family, a secure social position, power in the relationship – and female desire is denied and suppressed. This asymmetrical pattern in relation to the body has consequences for the gendered patterning of personal care.

Across all the agencies there was a shared understanding that women were assisted by female careworkers, and men by either female or, on occasion, male workers. Paulette Gibson, the manager of a not-for-profit agency, summarised the expectations: 'Women don't have men doing personal care and ... men are so used to women doing personal care [that] some men ... would rather have a woman do it than another man.'

When asked, most female respondents were clear that they did not want a male careworker, and some felt this strongly. Mrs Bucknell responded: 'Oh, no. I wouldn't have a man. No thank you!' But it is important not to assume that current modesty is necessarily a product of prudishness in the past. As Mrs Elster explained:

> I've lost most of my modesty, but I don't like the idea of a man seeing me naked, I'm of the old school. I wasn't a prude. In fact I liked fun and games in my time, but not now, no.

A small number of respondents were indifferent; for them accepting care had been the great change, and the gender of who gave it mattered little.

The asymmetrical pattern of tending was not, by and large, an issue within home care. Most agencies would not send a male careworker to a female client; and the possibility of this was anyway rare since the great majority of careworkers are female (as indeed are clients). The realities of recruitment and of demand thus deliver to agencies a pattern that is in line with dominant assumptions. As a result, care managers, while acknowledging the asymmetry, had rarely been required to consider its meaning. As Roz commented 'There's an unwritten rule about that and that's all I'm gonna say.'

The response of male clients to cross-gender tending was different in tone from that of women. They saw help from a woman as a normal part of gendered expectations; and they often presented it in a slightly flirty, nice-for-me, sort of way. (As we shall see women careworkers also used joking to negotiate the encounter.) For men, being seen and touched by a woman was potentially nice and carried none of the sense of threat that cross-gender touch might for a woman. As Jacqui explained:

> A lot of the men quite enjoy having a woman. And honestly I think, you know, specially a nice young girl come to help them have a bath, they like it. You know, not in any sort of perverted way, just, just in a you know, they like the attention.

Mr Wagstaffe concurred with this sentiment:

INTERVIEWER: Did you find it embarrassing at first or—?
MR WAGSTAFFE: Well not really. I thought it might be more embarrassing for *them* than for me, but they don't seem to mind a bit.
INTERVIEWER: Why did you think it would be more embarrassing for them?
MR WAGSTAFFE: Well, the first girl I had she was only about eighteeen I think. She was a sort of punk, she'd got bright red hair and earrings in her eyebrows. Sort of girl that a person of my age looks at and thinks Gawd Almighty. But she was absolutely sweet, she was a lovely girl. It turns out that they nearly all live with their boyfriends or something, so I don't bother about it now ... And young ladies in their early 20s these days are rather different from when I was the same age.

So he felt that any responsibility that he might have had for protecting the innocence of young ladies had been discharged.

Most of the men in the study had female careworkers, though a few had a man. The majority of these had not asked for a male worker. It had simply been a matter of making up rosters (though it can be a response to clients who misbehave sexually). Some men indeed dislike the idea of a same-sex careworker, perceiving it in terms of a potentially homosexual encounter (a feeling reinforced by their assumption that carework is not work for a proper man). As Mr Hedges, an older black man, made clear, he did not want a gay worker: 'I would not like a poofter now, they're different.... I don't want a poofter touching me at all.'

The only occasion in the study where a male careworker had specifically been asked for was by a gay couple. They did not feel at ease with intimate care from a woman. 'We have always asked for a male because we don't – we like women – but we don't, somehow we are not happy when they are bathing.' They wanted a man – though they repudiated any suggestion that they might prefer a gay man (perhaps as part of repudiating the sexuality of bathing itself).

MR KIRKWOOD: It would not occur to me.
MR BOYD: No, it wouldn't occur to me ...
MR KIRKWOOD: You don't think about it.

Some careworkers believed that male clients preferred a female worker not for reasons of sexuality, male or female, but of dominance. As Roz put it, 'I think sometimes men are more threatened by a man going in there than a woman, I think they can kind of, like push you more about, than they would dare to if it was a man carer going in.'

Age, gender, sex

There are reasons to think that the issue of cross-gender tending is more sensitive for younger recipients. This is not to endorse any sense that older people are asexual. It is clear that sexuality remains profoundly significant throughout people's lives; and as we have seen, people do not cease to care about exposure just because their bodies are no longer young and in conventional terms desirable. However, it was clear that for some younger people in the study, the issue of bathing raised very directly questions of sex. For Sharon Kimpson, a women in her early thirties with a young child and living with her mother also disabled, the fact that she is still of an age to have a sexual life was relevant to the embarrassment she felt about bathing. Her mother commented on her 'hang ups', which she – also receiving help – did not share. Sharon retaliated by attributing this to the fact that she is still of an age to be sexually active. Her mother agreed that she might have felt differently when she was younger (though she did not like being wholly pushed aside sexually). For both of them, the issue was linked to age.

MOTHER: I haven't got the hang-ups about it that you've got though.
SHARON: Yeah, but I'm younger than you, aren't I?
INTERVIEWER: So what would you feel – would you feel ...
MOTHER: I wouldn't take a lot of notice, it don't affect me really.
INTERVIEWER: Would you have felt that when you were younger as well, do you think?
MOTHER: Probably not.

SHARON: Yeah, but when you're young you're still sexually active, aren't you, you still look at men and think: 'Oh!'

MOTHER   *Excuse me,* I'm not that old – *excuse me!*

SHARON: Yeah, well you don't go on about it like I do. If there's something on telly ... I mean I said hello to a policeman the other day, I nearly dropped down – he said hello to me!

Tensions around the bounded nature of the intimacy arise most strongly where sexual intimacy is indeed a possibility. Paul Hubbard was a man in his thirties with cerebral palsy living independently in an adapted bungalow. He was very conscious of the danger of overstepping the mark. Some of the careworkers had been young, and he would like to give them a kiss, but he knew he must be careful; and he cited the example of a man he knew who was accused of brushing up against the careworker while at a residential centre and was then not allowed to go back to his home. As a result he was very careful how he behaved.

> I might like give em a kiss at Christmas, but then, if I ever did do anything like that, sexual harassment, God, I'd be jeopardising my place and – er, I've worked so hard to get this place – you know that would be terrible.

The actual process of bathing could be difficult because it could be sexually arousing. Sometimes he would masturbate afterwards, but never when they were there.

> I've never, I've never done anything like that when she's been like, in the, in the – helping me – like when she's gone shopping, if I've done that, I might have done that quickly, but I've never done it, like in front.

As hard as the directly sexual aspects were the problems of becoming too fond. One careworker in particular:

> I really liked, I really would've liked to, liked to have got to, like to, you know, more of a relationship, but she left and er, that was hard because we were on the same wavelength – cos we got well, had jokes together – she was a lovely person, yeah, I was, say cos I got, got attached to her, but then I knew that she, I had to tell meself that she was there just to help me.

Partly to counteract such feelings but also to establish the nature of the relationship in the interview, he tended to present his current careworker more in terms of a mother. 'She is like a mother – always sees that I'm all right in the bath and that and makes sure it's not too hot and that.'

Bounded intimacy

The physical intimacy of sex is a powerful factor in creating love and closeness within a relationship. Is there any parallel effect in relation to bathing? Does its physical closeness create a different, deeper sort of relationship than one where care is more circumscribed? Evidence from the study was equivocal, but did not by and large support such an interpretation. In the interviews, few of the clients or careworkers warmed to the idea. It was hard initially to assess whether this was because the hypothesis was fundamentally mistaken, so that the idea struck no chord in their experience, or because the constraints on talking about, even thinking about, this area were so strong. As we have noted, to verbalise pleasure in touch was difficult. Endorsing the idea of physical closeness as a means to other closeness seemed to imply an inappropriate sort of relationship.

The only person who did verbalise these aspects was Stella. She was relatively unusual among careworkers in that the main focus of her work was elsewhere, as a singer-songwriter, and she only did bathing work part-time as a source of money and other satisfaction. For her, the act of taking clothes off in front of another is a divesting the self of barriers, giving up your boundaries and opening the self to intimacy; this means that baths inevitably involve an intimate exchange.

> The actual act of in our society of getting your clothes off in front of somebody else is like so much more than just, than just the act itself, it's kind of like giving away your barriers and your boundaries and so what you're saying is almost like that what you say keeps up the front. What you do, the intimacy of what you do is real, the real real part.

Carework took place at a deeper and more intimate level than just the surface world of talk. This means that you need to be sensitive to boundaries.

> It's just intuition really but that's probably a bit of a vague word it's kind of knowing ... a boundary not to cross it ... when

somebody has a boundary not crossing it that you're not actually you know you have a task you're supposed to be doing something for them you can encourage and encourage and create, facilitate an environment that will make it so that they can do that but you never force anyone to do anything and you never out step the boundaries but at the same time you gently. I don't know it's like moving back and forth gently you're getting them to a place where they feel fully comfortable.

For her, the physical nature of the work brings you close to people in an intuitive way; and this applies even when you do not really know anything much about them. In her view, the closeness and intimacy of the work creates its own form of connection.

The majority of people in the study did not, however, see things this way. For many the physical intimacy was discordant rather than supportive. When Sharon, the young woman in her thirties, was asked if the physical closeness of bathing made for a closer relationship with the worker she replied: 'No, not really. No, in fact, probably the other way.' Her mother, who also received help, added: 'I think bathing is too personal to get friends, to make friends with someone that's doing the bathing – other ways, yeah, but not, not bathing.' Roz, a careworker in Coastville, similarly felt that the physical intimacy of bathing got in the way of the relationship. Bathing did produce a form of closeness, but not in her view a nice one. It was an enforced thing, that went beyond the boundaries that many people, including herself, felt happy with. Her colleague in the interview, Kathryn, did feel bathing led to greater emotional closeness, and that clients were more willing to confide in the worker and express their feelings, though she noted that this traffic was one-way.

> When they're in the bath, like to sort of tell you things ... they do say things that they possibly wouldn't tell their families you know, so we, we do get a lot of confidential little stories and little things that's happened in their lives, so they build up that relationship. But as far as we're concerned we don't have that same relationship with them, that's where it stops.

Roz however viewed this process more cynically. She believed that people in the bath are vulnerable, so that they blurt out secrets in an attempt to make up for their sense of unease. The giving of a secret is here is a form of offering to placate the person in the context where the recipient feels vulnerable and at a loss (a view that is supported by the literature on the links between embarrassment and compliance).

> It's true that when somebody's in the bath, they tell you things that they probably wouldn't when you were having a cup of tea ... I think it's to do with their embarrassment ... if I was sitting in the bath and somebody was talking to me that would probably be the time when I was feeling more vulnerable and so maybe I might say things that I wouldn't usually want to say.

In general therefore what people appeared to want in a bathing relationship was a form of intimacy, but one that was bounded in its nature. The closeness of bathing is not the same as the closeness of other forms of friendship, indeed the two are to large extent at odds, as the comments of Sharon and her mother show. Personal care is by its nature discordant; it sets up a series of dissonances around closeness, intimacy, distance, boundaries and roles, and these are played out in the care encounter. We can observe this also in the views expressed by older and disabled people about who should best give this care.

Who is best to do this work: families, friends, nurses, strangers?

Personal care can in theory be provided by a range of people: relatives, friends, auxiliaries, nurses, as well as careworkers. It is sometimes assumed that close kin will be the preferred source for personal care, and that the generalised norm that endorses seeking help from kin will apply all the more strongly where the care is of an intimate nature. Evidence from work with older people and their relatives, however, suggests that this is not necessarily so; and many older people prefer not to receive such help from kin. Daatland (1990) for example, found that in Norway (where public provision has high general acceptance), while two thirds of older people would prefer to look to public services for help with housework; when the issue was personal care, the proportion rose to three quarters.

Ungerson attributes such reluctance to the strength of the incest taboo which she describes as a powerful 'background noise' behind the day-to-day surface of informal tending (Ungerson 1983: 75). People are disturbed by activities that violate this norm; and personal care can literally mean uncovering a parent's nakedness. It proved difficult in the study, as Ungerson herself found, to get people in the talk directly about this; and most who found intimate care for an opposite-sex parent difficult, were unable or unwilling to expand upon their feelings: it was just something that they felt very strongly they did not want to do. Mrs Scott caring for her father explained:

MRS SCOTT: I couldn't bring myself to bath my dad.
INTERVIEWER: Why did you think that, why do you think that is?
MRS SCOTT: Well I suppose being a man and it was my dad.
INTERVIEWER: Yes sure.
MRS SCOTT: I mean I know when I went to see Dr. Baxter and I said to him – Don't ask me to do it, because I can't do it.

And she added: 'It is my dad and I can't. I mean I will do anything else for him.' Her father, a retired gardener, shared these feelings: 'I wouldn't have my daughter do it,' but could not be persuaded to elaborate. For one working-class woman in her eighties, the norm was so strong that she could not believe that the interviewer was seriously suggesting that her son might help her bath.

Careworkers and managers are familiar with these feelings. One London worker explained:

> I have a lady, she wouldn't let her daughter bath her. And Francine said to me, 'Toni, I can't understand why my Mum won't let me give her a bath.' I said 'Francine, you're her daughter,' but I understand, and she said to me, 'But you give her bath.' I said 'Look, I'm not, I'm a stranger. I've known your Mum for a lot of years. She trusts me more, to give her bath, because I'm a stranger, but because you're her daughter,' because she even said 'But, Mum, I know you're not a spring chicken anymore', she said 'No but you don't understand.' I do understand, because of the way she was brought up, you know. I'm a stranger, so that's alright for me.

I would agree with Ungerson that part of the particular charge around this area for kin does indeed relate to incest and to the dangerous qualities of that intimacy. The feeling is strongest in relation to parental tending, particularly for an opposite sex parent; and it is strongest of all in relation to sons caring for mothers, where there is the added aspect of transgressive activity for a male. But these feelings are also found – to a lesser degree – between couples, which suggests that the issue is not only one of threatening a 'non-sexual' parental relationship with a dangerous sexual intimacy. There were couples in this and an earlier carer study (Twigg and Atkin 1994) who preferred not to be involved in intimate care. Sometimes this included bathing, though more problematic were interventions that involved incontinence or bowel function. Parker found that many younger couples experienced intimate care as embarrassing and difficult; and though the carers tended to become inured to the situation, the recipients of care often remained unhappy about it. Parker concludes that we should not assume, as earlier work had, that intimate care between spouses is unproblematic and covered by the general rubric concerning the physical intimacy of marriage. The physical intimacy of sex is different from the physical intimacy of care; indeed the two can be at odds. Being cared for, particularly where it involves infantalising activities like washing, feeding, managing incontinence, can destroy the sexual element in a relationship, eroding the adulthood on which it rests, and at some level inevitably reducing the person in the eyes of the spouse and themselves. In Parker's study these feelings were expressed particularly strongly by the person receiving the care (Parker 1993, Parker and Seymour 1998).

This suggests that the difficulty with intimate kin care is not simply one of incest but lies in a more generalised threat to the relationship. What is done is important here. The difficulty centres around tending that involves a diminution of the person – wiping their bottom, washing the body, feeding them – care that erodes their status as an adult. What older and disabled people dislike about intimate kin care is their loss of status in the eyes of the person who is close to them. They fear that the person they were – and to themselves still are – will be lost. Similarly carers want to continue to experience their mother/uncle/sister as the person they always knew, and that by and large means someone with their clothes on, managing their own body functions and relating to them in a sociable way. It is a mistake to see intimacy as lying along a single continuum with strangers (least intimate) at one end and spouses (most intimate) at the other, and with physical and visual access graduated through. Though there is truth in this, it is too simple. Different sorts of intimacy pertain to different relationships.

If kin relations can be problematic in this area, what about friends? Not surprisingly the same difficulties apply. Friendship classically rests on reciprocity and equality; and changes that disturb the equality, threaten the existence of the friendship. As a result, friendship is rarely the basis for caring in any long term or serious way; and this applies particularly to intimate care which transgresses the normal physical boundaries of friendship. Sharon Kimpton had a friend who was a careworker and she asked as a favour since she was looking for work, if Sharon would ask her care manager to contract with her to do the bathing. But for Sharon this was a most unwelcome idea. Having a friend would be worse than anything. Lawler (1991) similarly found that pre-existing friendships made nursing difficult and potentially embarrassing.

By general agreement, the preferred source of such care was a stranger, or at least someone who had started out as a stranger, but had then become familiar. What people wanted was a relationship with the careworker, but one that was specialised in nature, particular to the activity of caregiving, offering warmth and closeness, but within a defined and bounded set of expectations.

One of the possible ways of balancing the need for care with the wish for distance is by using nurses to negotiate intimate care. Nurses are culturally sanctioned to perform such tasks, and the distancing techniques that they traditionally deploy – uniforms, professional manner – can, it has been argued, make the negotiation of bodily intimacy easier. This was not, by and large, how respondents in the study saw it. Few warmed to the idea of a nurse, and most preferred the relationship with an untrained careworker, and they felt at ease with what they saw as a warmer and more domestic relationship. Nurses were perceived negatively, as unreliable in relation to low level community care needs like bathing, and they often reminded older people of bad experiences in hospital where their bodies had been pulled about in the processes of illness, investigation and treatment. Abbott (1994) similarly argues that the claims of the community nursing service to be preferred by clients as a source of help with bathing is not supported by evidence from older people; and she interprets this emphasis on the special character of nurses by the profession as a form of occupational closure.

Lastly, some careworkers felt that bathing was best provided by a specialist worker who only gave baths, and that this best preserved the bounded character of the relationship. Mixing the cleaning of the house and the person in their view disturbed the special character of the relationship, implying a depersonalisation in which the elderly person becomes like the dishes or the floor, a thing to be cleaned. From the careworkers' point of view the issue was bound up in questions of occupational status. In relation to the recipients, it was certainly the case that the warmest relations in the study were with the specialist bathing service. There did seem to be a particular closeness there. How far this was the product of the specialist character of the service, as opposed to the personal qualities of the workers, is hard to assess. The workers certainly believed it was. As Stella commented: 'The intimacy couldn't be as intimate if that person was caring for you in all respects all the time.'

Conclusion

For most people in the study, receiving help with bathing and washing had been an unwelcome development in their lives. These are aspects of living that individuals prefer to manage for themselves; and indeed personal care is defined in terms of the self-care that adults, however wealthy or pampered, do for themselves. Crossing this boundary, therefore, marks a major shift in people's lives. Most respondents approached the issue with stoicism, recognising that these were changes that had to be accepted. A few still found the business embarrassing, but most had adjusted, and many had indeed come to welcome the help they received, throwing off their initial unease and taking pleasure in the experience. While bathing could never be quite what it had been, there was still some sensuous enjoyment to be had from it, and in the company of careworkers whom they liked, was a source of pleasure and human contact.

The experience of receiving help was an individual thing, though one strongly mediated by social and cultural expectations, particularly in relation to gender and age. Many older people have internalised a negative perception of themselves and of their bodies, and exposure particularly before staff who were young was a source of discouragement. We will see in Chapter 7 how the careworkers felt about this, and about how confronting aging bodies raised existential questions for them about their own futures. Gender was also a powerful factor mediating the experience, as we have seen in the conventions concerning cross-gender tending and the differential responses of men and women. In Chapters 6 and 7 we will explore the significance of these conventions from the perspective of the careworkers, looking at how such gendered patterns circumscribe the activities of male careworkers and contribute to the construction of carework as gendered labour. Lastly, receiving help with bathing is mediated through a special sort of relationship. By and large recipients prefer not to mix personal care with other sorts of relationship, notably kinship or prior friendship. The transgressive nature of the care means that it is at odds with such. Recipients prefer to receive such help from individuals with whom they have developed a specialised relationship, one that may involve friendship, emotional closeness and trust, but that is of its nature distinct and bounded.

4 The spatial and temporal ordering of care

Community care takes place in a special space – home – and a special time – that of domestic life. Time and space are two of the fundamental categories of social order, and it is within their matrixes that daily life, with its rhythms and regularities, takes place. One of the aims of this book is to reassert the significance of the ordinary and the mundane in the analysis of community care, and the spatial and temporal ordering of care are part of this. In this chapter we will explore the consequences for both clients and careworkers of the coming of care into the spatio-temporal world of home, looking in particular at issues of privacy, control and power. We will also explore a rival setting for bathing help – the day centre – showing how this reveals in reverse some of the central meanings of bathing at home.

Public and private

The distinction between the public and the private is fundamental to the spatial ordering of the home, though it operates in complex ways. Public and private do not sit neatly apart but are constantly intersecting and articulating with each other at a number of levels (Mason 1989). Two of these levels are of particular significance in relation to domiciliary care. The first is the opposition between the public world outside the home and the private within. The coming of care represents not just a crossing of that boundary, but the intrusion into the private world of values, rationalities and temporal structures that belong to the formal world of service provision. The second level concerns the overlapping contrasts between public and private space within the home itself. These structure and express social relations, and give form to daily life. Before we explore the significance of these spatial oppositions, however, we need to discuss the meaning of home more generally since this is a fundamental element in structuring expectations concerning privacy and space.

The meaning of home

A range of work, much of it phenomenological in character, has explored the social meanings of home (Lawrence 1987, Allen and Crow 1989, Sixsmith 1990, Gurney and Means 1993). Among these meanings, privacy is central. As Allen and Crow (1989) point out, the absence of privacy is one of the most disliked aspects of living in hostels or residential homes and central to the feeling that these are not really homes at all. Privacy depends on the physical capacity to exclude – to shut the door on the outside world. Friends and relations who visit the home do so on a privileged basis as guests. Restricting access to certain people and certain times allows you to maintain a socially appropriate 'front stage' and to conceal the ways in which your life falls short of the domestic ideal. This relates to a second feature of home, its association with relaxation and ease. To feel 'at home' is to be at your ease. Home is also, for most people, a place of security: a haven from the possibly harsh and threatening world outside; and this can be particularly significant for older people who may feel vulnerable outside their own territory. Lastly, home is a site of identity and self expression, an opportunity to extend the self in material surroundings. For many older people, home is particularly significant as embodying the memories of a partner; and its material surroundings are a daily remainder of continuity with past identity and relationships (Rubinstein 1989, Belk 1992, Gurney and Means 1993). By contrast, nursing homes are 'placeless spaces' in their uniformity of objects and rooms, their neutrality and lack of distinguishing or personal features (Rubinstein and Parmelee 1992). Home also anchors people within a locality, and even older people who do not go out retain a vivid local map and sense of their place within the wider community (Gurney and Means 1993).

In discussing the meaning of home, it is important to acknowledge that people's experiences are not always as positive as the ideology implies. Home can be a place of abuse and personal unhappiness – all the more so because of its privacy. For many women, it is a place of work as much as of leisure and ease; and for those without jobs to link them to the wider world, it can embody isolation and loneliness. Allen and Crow (1989) characterise the lives of many older people as not so much positively home-centred as negatively home-bound.

Many older people in the study were effectively imprisoned in their flats as a result of narrow and steep stairs, and they longed to get out; however this did not fundamentally affect their feelings about their homes which by and large remained positive.

The ideology of home is almost universally recognised and endorsed within British culture, and its principal features – the ethic of privacy, the power to exclude and the embodiment of identity – are significant in structuring the care encounter from both sides. These central values are as much endorsed by the careworkers as by the older and disabled people. Workers regard their own homes in the same way, so that rules of behaviour that attach to these values are part of the taken-for-granted reality of their own social lives. The 'power' of these structures is thus deeply embedded socially, and does not have to rest solely on an internalisation of 'good practice'. This is important in explaining the degree of power that home gives to recipients.

Crossing the divide: the private world of home

Careworkers, in entering the home, enter space that they recognise as private; and some described the uncertainty of the first visit, waiting on the doorstep wondering who and what lay behind the front door. 'The first time is always a bit, I mean I can feel, it's not my territory. And it's theirs, and I feel really not at ease.' Coming into the home of someone is an odd and unsettling experience, one that can make careworkers feel vulnerable. As Kathryn in Coastville explained:

> I think you feel a little bit humble as well, because you're going into a strange person's home, and even if they ask you to make a cup of tea, it's like going into your friend's house and your friend says, go and make a cup of tea, unless you've been in that friend's house before, you don't know where the cups are and you don't know where the sugar's kept, and it's sort of like you're in there in somebody's house as a worker ... it's a very, very weird experience.

Although they come to do a job of work, they accept that they are in some measure bound by the norms of being a guest. These mean that you have to ask permission both to enter and to do certain things. Some clients were very guarded about their space; others less so. As one careworker commented:

You can walk into a place that's like a palace and somebody will be very free with it and just let you wander around. You walk in somewhere that is in squalor and they'll be very precious about everything you touch.

Workers are bound by the general social norms of not being over-inquisitive or looking openly around and not going beyond limited permissions, particularly in the early stages of the relationship: 'You don't take anything for granted. I mean I wouldn't just go and get towels or anything.' Care staff were explicitly instructed not to wander about or look in drawers in case there were accusations about theft.

From the perspective of the clients, receiving help means having to accept people coming into the home. Responses to this varied, and class and gender were both relevant. Those with middle and upper-middle class backgrounds, accustomed in the past to having domestic help, in some cases servants, were unsurprisingly the least concerned about the potential intrusion of careworkers. Sir Peter, a retired senior naval officer, interpreted the experience positively:

INTERVIEWER: Do you ever mind all these people coming into your house?
SIR PETER: Not in the least.
INTERVIEWER: So you never feel it's a bit of an invasion of your—
SIR PETER: No, I was delighted.

Others did feel it an intrusion, though one that they simply had to accept as part of the cost of staying at home. For some the presence of any careworker in the home, particularly if unfamiliar, created a sense of unease. Mrs Sheils, living with her partner Mr Hedges, commented: 'You have to sit and, you know, there's a stranger in the house, and you feel, well, good, they'll soon be finished, and that will be it.' The ease of home had been disturbed by the presence of a stranger, and it could not be restored until they had gone.

For Mrs Bucknell it was more a sense that her life itself was now on view, open to public scrutiny and comment. Accepting careworkers for her meant that her home had become part of the wider public world outside. Though she could no longer get out, she remained very conscious of local reputation, and she was concerned that one of the careworkers was a gossip and felt that the whole world now knew her business: 'They come in, you see, they know everything … and they know my business, and everything – so I don't like it.'

Responses to the intrusion of care tended to reflect gender. The sense was more strongly expressed by women, unsurprisingly since women are more closely associated with the territory of home, and more accustomed to controlling and ordering it. Mr O'Brien, by contrast, an Irish working class man caring for a wife with dementia, was happy to hand over the space of the flat to the careworkers when they came to give his wife a bath and clean the flat.

MR O'BRIEN: I get to know them very well, yes. Of course, when they come here they're in charge of the flat, they're in charge of the kitchen, they can help themselves to whatever they want. I make it quite clear to them that the kitchen's there for them.
INTERVIEWER: So you hand it over to them, as it were?
MR O'BRIEN: Yes, entirely, yes, yes – oh yes, yes.
INTERVIEWER: And that's OK, you don't feel they kind of come bustling in and—
MR O'BRIEN: No, no, no, no – no, they're quite, quite good [used here as a positive emphasis].

For him, domestic territory was naturally female, and receiving help there in tune with normal gender expectations.

For Mr Colegate, however, the coming of help was experienced as an intrusion. He cared for a wife with MS and the steady progress of her disease meant that more and more of the space of the home was dominated by her care needs. Careworkers came and went all day. He sometimes had no sense of who would be in the house.

INTERVIEWER: Do you ever feel that your house is a bit taken over by all sorts of people from all these agencies I mean?
MR COLEGATE Well sometimes, I hate it, it doesn't feel like me own house, I've never really settled here to be honest.

As a defence he had instituted an informal reordering of the house, recasting the kitchen, where his wife no longer went, as an office-cum-sitting-room for himself. There at least he was able to establish some control over the space which was otherwise dominated by her care needs and the activities of careworkers.

The power of home

The ideology of home plays an important part in the power dynamics of care, endowing older and disabled people with an element of control, and making it possible in some degree to resist the dominance of careworkers and professionals. Home is space that belongs to the occupant, and this social norm is underwritten legally. Older people can refuse admission to professionals and shut the door in their face. Social services have no general powers of entry (even in the case of children), and short of 'sectioning' the individual, or making them subject to an order under the Public Assistance Act 1948 (something only done rarely when the conditions of the individual are so extreme as to threaten life), they cannot force their presence or their care on reluctant recipients. The strength of the legal position may not always be understood by clients, but the social norm on which it rests is. There were examples in the study where older and disabled people had exerted control over the situation and effectively 'dismissed' a careworker, asking that they should not be sent again. Though I would not want to exaggerate this element of control, it does ultimately rest on the capacity to exclude, that material and ideological feature of home. It is impossible to believe that older and disabled people would be able to exercise this kind of preference or control over staff employed in institutional settings.

The second source of power derives from the home as the embodiment of identity. This puts a limit on the degree to which an individual can be depersonalised. To be depersonalised is at worst to lose your name, your history, your identity; it is to be literally and metaphorically stripped, made subject to anonymous and collective regimes, the process classically described by Goffman (1961) in his account of the Total Institution. But at home, surrounded by your possessions – family photographs, pictures of yourself when young, holiday mementoes, books – it is not possible to be wholly reduced to anonymity. In this setting, it is hard for someone to be treated like a cypher, an object simply to be cleaned and ordered. The surroundings of home are therefore an important buttress of the individual. Mrs Ostrovski was a large powerful women with a vigorous mind who had worked as a translator, but who was now confined to her bed, camped out in the corner of a rambling flat filled with books, pictures and itinerant lodgers. She explained how personal possessions establish social status. This is important because being dependent is depressing, and possessions help you to maintain a sense of self. She contrasted this with what went on in hospital:

MRS OSTROVSKI: Because maybe at home, when you are at home and around all sorts of rubbish of yours so they don't think you are exactly, you know, bad you know, but in hospital you are just coming out of the crowd, you are aged seventy five – 'Yes dearie, yes darling, good show, jolly good.'[mimicking a silly patronising tone]

INTERVIEWER: Right, so do you think having home around you makes a difference?

MRS OSTROVSKI: Well yes I think it gives you the – it gives you, because to need somebody's help, it's already – you need to concentrate your strength not to go down, not to become depressed.

Later we returned to the theme:

INTERVIEWER: You said something about all the things around you, and as I sit here I can see, you know, all these books and pictures and things.

MRS OSTROVSKI: That gives you identity, as I say, and *you* are not at a disadvantage. I think in hospital you are at a disadvantage. You are just a nonentity who came from the street, you know, and you are treated as they please. ... Here you are not the one lost. The other person is coming from outside. ... If we are talking of who is up and who is down, you are up. You are on your own ground.

This aspect of power and control was endorsed by the careworkers also. As Zara commented, again drawing on the contrast between home and residential care:

Them being at home, they feel more confident. In their own surroundings. And it's like, not saying that I am an intruder, but it does, like I am a bit of an intruder so I have to do things the way they want it done. ... If they're in the residential home I have to do for them what *should* be done and what I think is good enough for them.

The power of home also underwrites a capacity to say 'no' to professional interventions. You are in a much stronger position to refuse medication or medical intervention if you are on home ground. In relation to pregnancy, part at least of the desire for home births derives from this sense of being in your own territory and therefore more able to resist professional domination. In a similar way, it is easier for people with mental health difficulties to refuse medication if they are living at home. In the days before community care, medication was commonly imposed in the hospital, though in the absence of a 'section', there was no legal basis for this: the social setting was sufficiently all embracing and all powerful to override such considerations. The shift to community-based care has made such practices difficult and exposed their lack of legal sanction. One of the community nurses in the study recounted an example of such resistance based on place. He had a patient who refused to have an enema.

> [She] just wasn't prepared to have them. It was her home and she felt she was in control. And I got back to the day hospital who'd referred her and they said, well she's never any problem with us. We just tell her it's time for her enema and she has it.

He felt at first that he looked foolish in the eyes of hospital colleagues:

> They thought that we were being quite inadequate about it, in that we weren't pushing hard enough. But it's all to do with that shift of power. The power was in this woman's hands and she, you know, she chose to exercise it.

The limited time that the careworker spends in the house is also significant in the dynamics of power. One of the classic features of a total institution is that inmates spend their entire lives there under the control of the staff. There are no periods when staff are absent, and it is as hard to establish private time as it is private space. In domiciliary care, careworkers are only there for part of the day, and that gives a tangential quality to their presence in the home. There are long periods of time when the domestic ordering of the home is solely in the hands of the occupant, and when personal order reasserts itself.

Lastly, for community-based careworkers, their place of work is another person's home. It is never their territory. As we have seen they have to ask permission to go and get the towels or move freely about the home. Though one or two workers had set up a cache of cleaning equipment, none had established space that could be said to be their own. The majority arrived and left with their cloths and materials. This contrasts with the residential home where the space belongs not to the residents but the staff. It is they who are in charge and they determine the rules. Significant areas of the residential home – offices, rest rooms, staff toilets – belong solely to them (Gubrium

1975). In the private space of home, however, workers cannot establish this sort of spatial exclusion and dominance. It is the other way round and it is they who have to ask permission to move about freely. As a group of careworkers in Coastville who had worked in both sectors explained: 'In a residential home they're in your environment, but when you go to their house, you're in theirs – it is quite different, you can't treat people the same.'

People in residential care have to have a bath whether they want it or not:

GILLIAN: Well, they're a bit bossy in residential homes, aren't they …
SUSIE: In a residential home you give them a bath—
GILLIAN: You can't be like that in someone's house—
SUSIE: No. If you've got a bath day then you have your bath whether you want it or not. Whereas in your own home, as I said to you, you can't – you can try and persuade them to do that, but if they don't wanna bath, they don't wanna bath, and there's nothing you can do except try and persuade them – it's their home, their territory.

It is important in discussing the power of home not to present too rosy a picture. Careworkers are not always circumspect in their behaviour, and the balance of power remains heavily in their favour. Most care recipients are frail and many have problems with eyesight and hearing, as well as mental confusion. Theft remains a recurring issue in domiciliary care, and other forms of abuse are also a possibility. Sites of care that are hidden from view should, of course, be a cause of concern if not active suspicion. However there are dimensions of the care encounter as it occurs at home that diminish the likelihood of abuse. We will discuss these more fully in Chapter 6 but only note here that the ideology of home is an important element in these.

Spatial ordering within the home

A number of theorists have explored the ways in which domestic space is structured, in particular how it is ordered along a public/private axis (Lawrence 1987, Allan 1989, Munro and Madigan 1993, Pearson and Richards 1994). Certain areas of the house are public, relatively open to strangers and guests; others are private, used only by those who live there. There is a privacy gradient in which halls are more public than sitting rooms, which are in turn more public than bedrooms. Though the exact nature of this ordering has altered historically, the basic pattern of public/private, Lawrence argues, has been present since the industrial revolution. He suggests that these public/private oppositions link to a series of other binary categories: front/back, clean/dirty, symbolic/secular, special/day-to-day, in which the parlour exemplifies the clean/front/symbolic/special and the kitchen the back/dirty/secular/day-to-day.

Within the spatial ordering of the home, the bathroom is semi-private space – less personally private than the bedroom, but still part of the semi-private upstairs zone. Bathrooms are now located by preference upstairs, separated from other forms of washing and cleaning which take place downstairs at the back of the house. Strangers may 'visit' the bathroom but only on licence. The privacy derives partly from temporal factors relating to the way in which the home operates during the periods of time (for example bedtime) when strangers are not present; and spatial ordering is here linked to temporal ordering. It also derives from the bodily privacy that bathrooms imply. Bathrooms and lavatories are the only rooms in the modern house that have a door lock. People using them either do so alone or in the company of intimates. As Higgins comments in relation to institutional care, it is the bathrooms, toilets and bedrooms, areas which are normally considered intimate or private space, that 'become some of the most public rooms where personal territory and dignity are frequently invaded' (Higgins 1989: 168).

Re-ordered lives

Disability and its consequences threaten the traditional ordering of the home, in some cases imposing a radical reordering. In the study, this applied most strongly to those who were severely disabled and lived alone. In two cases this meant living one's entire life on or in the bed, that had become the total living space. In other cases, it was more a question of skills that would enable them to continue living at home and to some degree order their space in a traditional way. Here the internal contrasts of private and public were by and large maintained, though somewhat blurred. Careworkers were relatively free to move between these territories. Some part of their role was to assist the older person in maintaining the structure of what Goffman termed front and back stage (Goffman 1969). Careworkers here took on a liminal character working across the social boundaries: work in the bedroom and bathroom enabling the person to be presented clean and dressed in the sitting room. There was not always an audience for this, but it maintained morale and a sense of the proper structure of life.

I will explore these themes in greater detail by looking at two contrasting examples: Mrs Elster, where the order of the house was radically reordered around care, and Mr Hedges and Mrs Sheils where the traditional order was strongly defended and maintained. Mrs Elster is totally confined to her bed. She lives, sleeps, washes, dresses there. As she says: 'I've been sitting here like this for six years.' By the bed she has an elaborate set of tables on which are arranged all her needs: books, papers, pills, cushions. She has a stick to reach objects, and she also uses this to haul her legs up and manoeuvre them on to the bed when she wants to lie down. She has a chemical toilet next to the bed, and careworkers bring basins and cloths, so that the bathroom is brought to her and arranged around her body.

Her life has become condensed around the bed, and from this vantage point she commands the flat. Her control extends even to cooking and gardening. She has food and plants brought to her and she chops and sorts them on a table, replanting pots and dicing vegetables:

> I have the girls bring in on a large tray what is left in the fridge, not milk and that kind of thing, but food, eatables, perishables and then I pick over that. Well now, I would say to them, oh yes do this you see and also I will have a, what's the name, bread board and a small saucepan please.

She looks out into the basement space at the front of the high Victorian Italianate house and sees the plants and flowers. Social life is limited but she can wave at those neighbours who see her, though this only happens at twilight when her lights are on and the curtains are not drawn.

Maintaining this regime requires considerable mental effort. She has a complicated set of practices, and she orders herself and the flat closely: 'Because my routine is a little bit like a plan you know, general's plan of his army, got to do that, so we can do this, and if we don't do that, then we can't do that.'

She constantly thinks ahead. By dint of this and her determination and courage she has been able to remain at home for six years in difficult circumstances. But to do this she requires the help of careworkers, and they have to follow her directions closely. This can be a source of difficulty as they tend to resent such close ordering of their work:

> They don't like it, being told, although I try and do it as nicely as I can. Like today I, somebody doing something and I, what did I say, oh no not that, and she said [imitates someone making squealy niggly reluctant sounds].

Her immobility however enables them to escape, and they can use the space against her. She described how they hid in the kitchen, pretending to be working, while they called their friends on their mobile phones. They thus establish their own private territory in her flat, out of sight of her managing gaze.

We now turn to the opposite extreme, where the traditional ordering of public and private was fully maintained and careworkers closely restricted where they could go. This is most characteristic of situations where there was another family member living in the house and Mr Hedges and Mrs Sheils were the clearest example. Mr Hedges was disabled and lived in a rather dark housing association basement flat. A former hospital porter, he had come to Britain from the Caribbean in the 1950s. His partner, Mrs Sheils, was white. They both had a strong sense of the territoriality of the flat and of the parts of it that were private. As Mr Hedges commented: 'This lady [Mrs Sheils] has two places don't let nobody go – in the bathroom and her kitchen.'

This ordering of space even applied to close family like grandchildren. He did not mind a stranger coming in to help, provided they did not attempt to go anywhere they liked: 'There's certain place they can go, but certain place nobody, where I don't like – in our bedroom or our kitchen or anything – no way – not even our own children do it.'

When the careworker came to give him a bath, the clean clothes were laid out in the bathroom, so there was no need for the careworker to wander about looking for things in the bedroom, and he did not go into that space:

> My clothes is out, ... hung on the door inside the bathroom – when I bath he can just take them up. So we have no problem there. Anybody want to come here can come, but they must know what their place is, because if they don't, then they know where the door is.

Unusually in the sample, Mr Hedges was always dressed when the careworker arrived – most people wait in their night clothes – again part of maintaining normal life and its proprieties. It was notable that this pattern even applied to Joshua, the careworker with whom Mr Hedges was close. They had a lot in common, including the experience of being 'black' and coming to Britain as young men. Mr Hedges spoke of him warmly 'like a son', one of the few people in the study to use a familial model for the relationship. Even this closeness, however, did not erode the structures of privacy, and Joshua did not move freely about the flat.

Much of the strength of these structures related to the fact that Mr Hedges and Mrs Sheils were a couple. The spatial ordering of the house is linked to the structural intimacy of the couple. The capacity of couples to assert their privacy against helpers and professionals is an added dimension of the power of home. Home is a power base for older disabled people containing both ideological and material resources that can underpin their independence and power of self determination. This is strengthened in the case of couples who are better able to assert their privacy against the intruding eyes and judgements of workers and professionals. (This barrier applies also to the process of research itself. It proved hard to ask questions about intimate care in the presence of the other member of the couple. To do so became a violation of their own privacy and the partner typically put up a barrier that was not present when the disabled person was interviewed alone.) This is one of the reasons why couples pose difficulties for institutional care. A number of studies have noted the way institutions discourage the development of any physical relationships between residents (Wilkin and Hughes 1987). In large part this arises from negative attitudes to sexuality among the old. But it also reflects a recognition that the existence of a sexual, marital relationship creates a territory of privacy in which workers feel it awkward to intrude. The bedroom of a couple is private in a way that no other residents' can be. Although in theory single residents have their own private space, this is in practice constantly trespassed upon. In the case of a couple, however, the dominant norm is sufficiently strong to create unease and embarrassment even among care staff.

Alien spaces: baths at day centres

We now turn to the ways in which these ideas of public and private find their reversal in attitudes to bathing at a day centre. The idea of having a bath at a day centre was almost universally rejected by respondents – often in vehement terms. For some the very idea was abhorrent, and for most it held little appeal. The reason lies in the themes discussed above. Baths in a day centre represent the reversal of all that gives domestic bathing its meaning. Bathing at a day centre is a private act in a public place. An activity that is normally undertaken in private, in the part of the house that is reserved for the inhabitants, is transposed to a public space where people come and go, and in a setting that would normally be regarded as outside.

Part of the resistance to a day centre bath is dislike of the bother of getting dressed and undressed yet again, and in a sample with disabilities this is a serious consideration. But resistance to undressing is more than just to the inconvenience and effort. It is also about resistance to the idea of unwrapping the self in a public place. Getting dressed to go out involves the preparation of a street persona and presence. For some in the study, maintaining a proper appearance was a source of self esteem and something worth working at. Mrs Fitzgerald who had suffered very distressing and disfiguring operation scars said:

> I don't like my body any more, I don't like anybody else to see it, but if I can dress properly and, you know, and I can put stockings on and I've still got decent legs and get away with it – but I know I'm getting away with it, I know it's not true – ... a hoax, yes. But I can get away with it, but a lot of trouble.

Having a bath at a centre means dismantling this public persona, and not in the security of home. As a manager of home care explained, most clients see going to a day centre as a social event, a day out and prefer to dissociate it from problems with personal care.

Baths at day centres were regarded as semi-public acts. The space was not secure and there was a sense of being on show. 'You might as well sell tickets,' Mr Kirkwood, an upper-middle-class man, commented disdainfully. Day centres did not offer the security of home. 'You don't know what you are letting yourself in for,' he continued. They are busy places where people come in and out. Respondents conveyed a sense of unease that they might be intruded upon at any moment. As Mrs Colegate, a middle aged woman with MS, said in contrasting a bath at home with one at the centre:

> It's nice sort of privacy in your own home sort of thing, cos I find a place like West House, doors don't get locked which, it's a

good idea I suppose, but people wander in and if you're laying prostrate on, with nothing on and the door's opened and somebody, a total stranger's standing there, can be a bit, you know.

In this uncertain context, it is difficult to relax. This is particularly important because it undermines one of the primary potential advantages of a bath at a centre. Day centre baths because of their more elaborate equipment are able to provide 'proper baths', lying down, fully under the water, able to move with freedom and ease. But if the social reality is one of unease, in which you get the process over as quickly as possible, these pleasures are lost.

Day centre baths are found in a variety of venues. Some are provided in specialist health service units with white tiles, elaborate equipment and a technico-medical feel. Others, such as those in voluntary sector centres, can be more makeshift, but still with the feeling of the laundry room or utility space. Whatever the venue, there is an inherently clinical feel to them, with their pipes and drains, levers and hoists. This accentuates the alienating quality of the experience. The space is not domestic and comforting, it is medical and hard. As Mr Wagstaffe commented: 'I'd rather go into a car wash.' The manager at a day centre for people with dementia where they did give baths acknowledged that there can be problems where the bath looks 'like a space ship'.

This mechanical quality was present also in the account of Mrs Colegate who had experienced a bath in a specialist centre, and she conveyed both the sense of vulnerability it produced and the alienating quality of the experience of being exposed and washed down in the shower trolley:

> Well it's like a bath, it's in plastic and, well you're laying down you know what I mean, and they shower you on it and then its got a drainage hole one end ... You feel a bit vulnerable cos you're laying flat on your back, but it's quick, it's quick and it's thorough.

There is a sense here of making the person into an object to be washed, to be hosed down in the trolley. This alienating aspect is potentially present whenever people are taken and washed by others, but much less so in the setting of home, where domestic surroundings and personal associations weaken the effect.

Lastly, for some the idea of a day centre bath itself suggested an unwelcome collectivism and a promiscuous social mingling. One well-off women caring for an elegant 81 year old mother (black leotard, gold slippers, white carpet, glass tables) reacted strongly to the idea of a day centre bath:

DAUGHTER: I don't think my mother would go to a day centre and have a bath – *no way*.
INTERVIEWER: No, well that's interesting to hear the view, because obviously everybody's different.
DAUGHTER: What! municipal bathing, is it?
INTERVIEWER: No.
DAUGHTER: It sounds *dreadful* to me.
MRS FORSYTHE: That would be the last straw.

Shortly after, in the context of more general talk and after having mulled the subject over in parallel, the daughter interjects

DAUGHTER: Listen, I don't even have a shower in the gym when I go up – I wouldn't dream of using the showers round there. They've just spent a hundred thousand quid on the place.
INTERVIEWER: Really?
DAUGHTER: I think it's very demeaning to people when they get older to think that they don't have their dignity and their pride and should suddenly be divested of all that because they don't have the mobility or are unable to get around – I'm absolutely against that sort of treatment. It smacks to me of authoritarianism and I don't like it, I don't like it at all.

The daughter ran her own business and had strong private-sector values. The day centre bath for her represented an authoritarian collectivist ethic that she abhorred. Keeping oneself apart, especially from the low-status social groups who used public provision, was important for her. Mr Wagstaffe expressed similar feelings when he said in the context of day centre baths:

I'm not very potty about these public places, that's why I never used to use swimming baths or something like that. I used to think I don't want to go in there after all the small boys have gone in a piddled in it in the morning. Well that's how it is. ... I don't really like using public lavatories.

As Douglas (1966, 1970) has argued, the treatment of the bodily margins – whether in relation to washing, excreting or eating –

cannot be analysed in isolation from other margins. Comments about pollution, attitudes to dirt, anxieties about bodily mingling, are expressive of other, more social concerns. For some respondents, baths at a day centre operated in this context, threatening social exclusivity and undermining attempts to keep oneself apart from the polluting contact with the general public and its dirt. They represent the very reversal of the meaning of home with its ethic of particularity and individualism and its capacity to control and exclude strangers.

The temporal ordering of care

The last decade has witnessed an upsurge of interest among social scientists in the phenomenon of time. This work builds on philosophical developments earlier in the twentieth century particularly associated with the work of Bergson that emphasised the lived nature of time, locating this within a wider phenomenological account of being (Bergson 1910, Adam 1995, Urry 1996). Among historians, E.P.Thompson's seminal 1967 essay on time and the work discipline has spawned a mass of work on the rise of clock time and its significance in the creation of industrial society. Some of the current interest within social science relates to debates about globalisation and postmodernity, and to the sense that under the impact of new modes of communication time and space have been compressed, collapsed into one another (Harvey 1989, Giddens 1991). My concern here is less with these issues than with the perception of the plural and complex nature of time as it is experienced in the social world; of the different sorts of time and how they mesh or do not mesh in the care encounter.

Accounts of the plural character of time typically start from a critique of the hegemonic character of clock time (Adam 1995). Clock time emerged in the early modern period with the development of mechanisms of exact measurement, and with them the sense of time as abstract measurement rather than as the sequence of events or seasons. Unlike the variable rhythms of nature, the invariant, precise measurement of clock time is a human invention. Clock time is time created in the image of a machine: repetitive, sequential, measurable, homogeneous. Almost infinitely divisible into equal spatial units, a minute or an hour or a day (as measured by the clock, though not by the heavens) is invariant. Experiential time by contrast varies in its tempo: it flies or drags. Clock time tracks and measures motion; it is time perceived as space; but is itself indifferent to change. This is the time of science and – in idealised form – of industrial production. Time that is abstract and decontexualised, and that allows for the measurement, control and commodification of the labour process. It is the time that Taylorism rests on, and that created the world in which 'time is money'. Societies that rest heavily on clock time are societies where time efficiency, time budgeting and time management are central.

This humanly created time has been reified in modern society so that its artificial quality is no longer perceived. It has become natural. It constitutes the taken-for-granted reality in terms of which we live; with the result that we find it difficult to see the complex ways in which time operates in modern society. We become able to grasp Other Time primarily through the medium of exotic societies or past historical periods; and accounts of time often rest on false dichotomies that oppose traditional and modern, early modern and industrial, cyclic and linear. These suggest that while Other Time characterises the past or distant societies, modern life is lived exclusively in the realm of clock time. But Adam argues this is not so. Perceptions explored in relation to other societies apply to ours also, it is just that we have lost the capacity to articulate them. Clock time, rather than being the standard against which Other Time is constructed, should be understood as a socially and historically distinct form of time: one that emerged in the west and that has become dominant, but that coexists with other forms of time in modern consciousness. Time is not monolithic: past and future life, the body and its rhythms, routines, cyclic time, linear time, the time of aging and of birth, bells, clocks, planetary rhythms are all part of the multiple times that interpenetrate and permeate our life worlds.

There is no single, comprehensive taxonomy of times, but three broad forms are of significance in the analysis of community care: body time and the related domestic time; process time or the time of caring; and the clock time of economic production as embodied in service provision. It is the intersection of these different forms of time that create many of the conflicts and difficulties of community care.

Body time and domestic time

Body time is one of the most taken-for-granted dimensions of our daily existence, but also one of the most profound. The physiological processes of our bodies are temporally organised and orchestrated, so that our lives are permeated by rhythmic cycles: neural pulses, heart beats, cycles of the day, month and seasons. The body's circadian rhythms which are fundamental to our physiology, structure the day and night, so that even though we now have the means, through light and heat, to extend, alter and completely reverse this pattern, there are limits to the body's adaptability, and repeated and radical disruption leads to distress and ill health. Time as experienced on a day-to-day basis at the level of our bodies is a fundamental source of rhythm, order and wellbeing in our lives.

These bodily processes are contained within social structures: the round of the year, the seasons, week, the day. Social time is multiple and local, embedded in work patterns, social relations, cultural assumptions: the academic year, the cycle of the church, the holiday season, Friday after work drinks, Saturday shopping. It is the intersection of body time with these social structures that creates the domestic ordering of time. This structures the day-to-day flow of experience, just as the spatial ordering of the dwelling structures the home. Body servicing plays a major part in this. To a considerable degree, days are structured around the care of the body: getting up, dressing, washing, eating, excreting, sleeping. These form the bedrock of domestic life.

Eating provides a particularly clear example of this intersection of body and social time. Bodies need periodically to be fed (roughly every three hours according to the digestive cycle), but few people eat solely at the prompting of appetite. Eating is socially structured and the pattern of meals is commonly used to mark out the divisions of the day: time for lunch, too early for a drink, past supper time. Meals and eating are also the basis of significant social encounters. Meals are inherently social events and through the operation of commensality build up and reinforce relationships; and as such they play a central role in social reproduction, particularly of relations of gender and family (Charles and Kerr 1988, Murcott 1982). Their patterning and the way in which they punctuate the day are central in creating the rhythm and form of domestic life.

Similarly, sleeping and waking mark the division between days; and going to bed, getting undressed, falling asleep, arising to the new day, are all culturally defined acts. Elias's account of the civilising process charts the shift from a medieval world where the space in which sleeping occurred was commonly shared to one of increasingly specialised rooms; from sleeping naked to the arrival of clothes for bed; from sharing beds as the norm to expecting to sleep alone or only as a couple. With this process the bedroom – like the bathroom – becomes more private, and sleeping like other body functions is shifted behind the screens of private life. This marking of the time through special clothes is extended also to the day. There are garments and ways of dressing that pertain to private life in the home: dressing gowns, slippers, wandering about in semi-undress. These are forms that belong to the times when the house is closed to the public, and they are part of the temporal structure of privacy that parallels the spatial one discussed earlier. The coming of care potentially disturbs and disrupts these structures as it does spatial ones, and careworkers find themselves pitched directly into the intimacy of people's private lives.

Other body responses like excreting are less clearly defined socially in their pattern, and tend to be treated fairly freely as a response to body needs. The major exception to this is institutional life. Many old people in residential homes or hospitals are toileted at set times. It is a measure of the extent and rigidity of the time ordering in such places that this aspect of life, normally freely structured, is made subject to order. There are parallels here with the regimes of bodily control described by Goffman (1961) and Foucault (1977) in relation to prisons and other Total Institutions.

Washing and bathing similarly mark out the structure of time. Baths and showers are often used by individuals to mark transitions between social states and times of day. They are a personal and individual version of the rites of passage that as we have seen are frequently linked to the symbolism of washing and bathing. For example, people often have baths or showers at the start or end of the day. This is obviously convenient in terms of dressing and undressing, but it is also part of marking the shift between the states of sleep and waking at an experiential, bodily level. Some people have a shower when they get back from work, using that to mark the passage from the world of work and home, taking off their formal office clothes and washing away the cares of work. One respondent, Sir Peter, used to bath twice a day, when he got up and again in the evening before he changed to join his wife for drinks before dinner. Baths are also used as rites of passage in preparation for social events like parties. They were very commonly used in the recent past in Britain to mark the passage of the week: Friday or Saturday night representing bath night, and a number of older respondents recalled such patterns in their own lives.

The domestic ordering of time and the quiet satisfactions it could bring was well conveyed by Mrs Bucknell, the widow of a builder, who had herself been in service. Though she could only move about with difficulty, she still marked out her week in terms of domestic tasks, dusting objects, wiping down surfaces, and she derived quiet pleasure from ordering the rhythm of her day, largely punctuated by meals and by dressing and undressing:

> I potter about. As I say, in the morning after [the careworkers] go, they go about half past eight and that, then I get me, I get ready for me dinner. Well, today I've had minced lamb, well, in that I put carrots and onions and celery, and everything – and I thoroughly enjoyed it and I had and she got me a savoy, I had some greens and potatoes, and I made a ... pudding – anyhow, I made that and then after that, oh, I did some sorting out of some papers then I did some Christmas cards and got them sorted out – so it took me right up to dinner time – and then I had my dinner washed up, then I come in here and here I stop, then I go out and get my tea. Then I come in here again until 8.30 pm when Ann comes, [I sit in front of TV in dressing gown] and then, after that, I go into bed at 10 o'clock.

Process time, and the gendered time of carework

Process time was developed by Davies (1984) to describe the particular nature of carework, and the concept is rooted in Scandinavian work on care, particularly Waerness's (1987) concept of the rationality of caring. Carework is seen as having a different logic to that governing other – usually paid – work in society. Caring is work that puts the needs and feelings of care recipients to the fore, rests on empathy, and responds not to abstract rules or principles but the specifics of the situation. 'Needs are frequently unpredictable. The relation on which care is premised often requires continuity, and a form of time that is not primarily determined by a quantitative and abstract conceptual measurement. Care requires process time.'(Davies 1994: 279). Process time means: 'letting the task in hand, or the perceived needs of the receivers of care, rather than the clock, determine the temporal relations'(ibid.: 281). Davies gives the examples of feeding a baby or older person, or thinking about and visiting a friend in hospital, where it is hard to predict how long such actions will take. They take the time they take; and they are difficult to schedule or measure. Their boundaries are fluid; it is not clear exactly when they begin or end; and there is often a element of waiting, as well as of weaving together of several activities simultaneously. Process time is thus different from task-oriented time, which separates the task from its context and is ruled by the logic of the clock.

Many of the features that Davies describes in the context of carework are characteristic of women's lives and work more generally, and some feminists have argued that time itself is gendered in that it is experienced and constructed differently by men and women. Female time, Hantrais argues, is characterised by plurality and interdependence; it is a product of the interweaving and interconnection of different times: biological, social, chronological, processual, cyclic, linear. Clock-based concepts of time fail to capture the complex interplay of times that arises from the plurality of women's lives (Hantrais 1993, Leccardi and Rampazi 1993). Different times are accorded different status; and the times that are governed by commodified work time take precedence over those outside that time economy. Research on women's caring and emotional work, both in relation to informal care and paid carework, demonstrates how times which are not convertible into currency remain unvalued and often outside analysis. The richness of feminist accounts, which embrace both conscious and unconscious levels, Leccardi (1996) argues, come from their recognition of these different sources of temporal meaning. These ideas find further echoes in the work of Irigaray and Cixious whose watery metaphors present the fluidity and flux of women's bodies, experiences and language, and the ways in which these lead them to emphasise context and connectedness (Game 1995). This endorses a perception of female time as flowing, experiential and subjective as opposed to rigid and abstracted. Adam (1995) endorses such accounts of women's time which she sees as exemplars of time lived, given and generated in the shadow of the hegemony of clock time, but she argues that its features do not belong exclusively to women. All who are outside the time economy of work relations – unemployed and older people as well – know something of this world of Other Time. Men too, even when in the mainstream economy, experience the complexity of different and competing times.

The time of economic production

Central to Davies' analysis is the conflict between the process time of careworkers and mothers – her study was based on a nursery – and that of formal employment, the classic clock time of industrial production and the labour process. As we have noted this concept of time is hegemonic, and one of the purposes of this section of the book has been to question its dominance and explore aspects of time of greater relevance to the care encounter. However there are important ways in which clock time is significant in understanding domiciliary care. Care agencies to a large extent operate within this time context, or experience pressure from purchasers to do so. Domiciliary care is increasingly managed through time allocation. Care managers purchase or allocate units of home care time as least as much as they allocate or purchase tasks. The privatisation of care services and the purchaser/provider split have reinforced this tendency. Staff in care agencies increasingly work to time schedules that specify the time each task should take and the point at which they should move to their next client. Similar developments have occurred in community nursing services. As we shall see these concepts of time are potentially in conflict with time as ordered domestically.

Conflicting times: the time of old age and the time of carework

The recipients of domiciliary care are predominantly old. They no longer live their lives within the time economy of work. Like leisure or free time, the time of old age is constructed against the dominant status of paid work. Old people are time rich. But they know that their time does not have value in the way that a worker's does. Their time is *not* money. There is a incommensurability between the time of clients and of paid workers, and this fact has been a fundamental stumbling block in attempts to give economic value to the time spent by clients waiting, for example, for the careworker, or GP or hospital consultant. It is only in an artificial way that their time can be accorded money value. The social reality is that their time is free – in both senses of the word – and does not have a value in monetary terms. Furthermore though the time of the workers does have such value, care recipients do not by and large pay for it, but receive it in an unequal exchange, and this weakens their moral claim on it.

These understandings are important in structuring the care encounter. Recipients are aware that careworkers are pressed for time, and they try not to hold them up. Mrs Napier made a point of having everything laid out ready before the careworkers came, and she knew that she must not delay them with invitations for coffee, much as she might like to. Time for many clients is unending and fluid: often there is no other event in their lives until the next care encounter. But for the workers, time is pressing. They live in the context of clock time, with schedules to meet and tasks to be accomplished. For the careworkers, leaving older and disabled people, many of whom are lonely and isolated and who rely on them for human company, is one of the hardest aspects of the job.

Tensions also arise when the world of service delivery attempts to map its logic on to domestic life. Nurses sometimes encounter difficulties with patients who delay and re-schedule their medicine because its diuretic and other effects disturb the normal pattern of their day. Scientific medicine measures out the hours exactly, but domestic time moves to a different rhythm. The conflict between the rationalised world of formal services and the day-to-day lives of individuals is particularly visible in relation to body time; and the needs of the body present recurring problems for service delivery. Some care needs, typically shopping and cleaning, can be condensed or saved up, so that they can be responded to in a 'lump', at a time that suits the agency and with efficiencies of scale. Other needs can be scheduled fairly easily – for example help with getting up – though this demands that the person agrees to do so at a set time rather than variably and at will. Such needs however typically require frequent interventions if the help is to come at times that coincide with the expectations of domestic time for example in regard to meals. Other bodily needs however – going to the toilet, managing continence – are not predictable or regulatable. Yet other needs arise not from body processes themselves but from threats that may arise in conjunction with them: slipping on the stairs, falling ill and not being able to drink. These pose a different set of time problems. They occur in time, but not at set or predictable times. The passage of time after they have occurred is highly significant in defining their seriousness and can be recognised in advance, but the precipitating moment can occur at any time. These needs can only be met fully by constant surveillance.

Isaacs and Neville's influential 1976 account of long, short and critical interval needs was an attempt to capture some of these features for research and classificatory purposes, but it did not address the full complexity of the situation. In order to do this it is necessary to recognise that we are dealing not just with one, but a plurality of times. Body time is different from the clock time of industrial production or of science. It cannot be measured out, cut, put together, abstracted in the way that clock time – and to some degree service time – can be. The needs of the body cannot be saved up and dealt with once a week. This is time that stops and starts in an arbitrary way. The time of domestic crisis only starts ticking once the old person has slipped on the stairs. It is the disjunction between these forms of time and logic of service delivery rooted in clock time that causes many of the tensions in community care, and we shall return to this when we look at the rationalisation of home care.

Controlling time

Baths and showers in ordinary domestic life take place at the will of the individual, and last as long as they desire or can spare. Accepting help inevitably means losing some of this spontaneity and control, and baths become subject to a new and external form of time discipline. The London bathing service allowed fifty minutes for a bath; but in Coastville home care the rostered time was shorter, and some careworkers attempted to get through their work at an even faster pace. Mrs Gray, a middle-aged woman with breathing problems, recounted how one careworker:

> was going in and out of the house in quarter of an hour. And in that time, I'd had a bath and was washed and dressed. By the end of that quarter of an hour I was quite a limp rag ... She does take 25 minutes now, because I complained.

Even where the worker did not rush the activity, recipients were often conscious of the need not to take too long, valuing the time of the worker above their own pleasure. As Mrs Fitzgerald commented:

> I mean I don't expect to lie there and soak.... I don't do that because of her time. I would *like* to. But if any time she came in and said that she wasn't so busy I would say, you know: 'May I have a little soak?' It's just purely psychological, isn't it? ... I take as little time as I possibly can.

This sense of being rushed and of time pressure is particularly important because one of the valued aspects of baths is the sense of timeless space that they can offer in people's lives. Mrs Napier described how baths had been like this for her in the past in what had otherwise been a busy time-pressured life as a buyer in a department store. It was:

> very, very pleasant, relaxing more than anything. Because I al-ways did everything at the double, I never did anything slowly. So I would unwind, I'd get in the bath and think well I'll have to stay still for half an hour perhaps or more.

Once baths are no longer wholly under the control of the recipient this aspect of bounded free space is hard to maintain.

Lateness and unreliable time keeping are long established problems in the literature of community care (Sinclair *et al.* 1990). One of the most common complaints about bathing and personal care in the past has been the unreliability of the service: staff come late, if they come at all. This is particularly trying in relation to personal care where, if the worker fails to come, the client is left in limbo, unable to get on with the next stage of the day. Uncertain timekeeping is also a message about power. Someone who is habitually late conveys the message that it is their time that matters; and to wait on someone's presence is to be subordinate.

In the study, though there were one or two complaints about having had to wait, or of unreliability in the past, they were the exception. The majority of respondents said that they experienced no problems over timekeeping or reliability. This puzzled me, since previous studies had recurringly identified this as a problem. Three factors explain this. The first is the low valuation put by older people on their own time, referred to above. The second is the way in which lives have become re-ordered around care, and I will explore this more fully below. And the third concerns actual changes in the service world that mean that timekeeping has in fact become more reliable. In the past the district nursing service was the main provider of bathing help. For community nurses bathing was a residual category of work, something typically fitted in at the end of a shift when the other more acute work had been covered, and even where given by auxiliaries they had low priority. As a result, staff were frequently running late, unable to promise to get to the person that day, uncertain when it would be possible to come again. Now baths are predominantly provided by either dedicated staff, rostered to give a bath, or by home care workers. In both cases giving a bath has priority within their work. This shift of responsibility appears to have affected the quality of time keeping.

The re-ordering of time

No one in the study received a bath in the evening, and this was despite the move to a more fragmented service that in theory allowed for interventions throughout the day. In earlier work I suggested that such restriction in relation to timing was likely to be disruptive in people's lives and disliked by them (Twigg 1997). As we have seen, baths are meaningful. People use them as rites of passage through the day, and being forced to undergo one at a meaningless time is thus potentially disjunctive. But the interviews did not by and large bear this out. The majority of people were happy with the pattern of provision. The key to this lies in the changes that had occurred in their own lives.

Many respondents had effectively re-ordered their lives around care, imposing a new temporal order in parallel to the spatial one discussed earlier. Many were very disabled; they lived alone and could not get out; and for them the conventional structure of the day had no great relevance. They were no longer linked into those patterns. (This was in contrast to younger and less disabled recipients or those who lived with others. For these individuals punctuality and timing in relation to the service remained important.) In so far as these more disabled recipients related to time structures, they were those rooted in the formal care system itself. Time for them had become reordered around the schedule of care. Thus Mrs Stanhope, when asked if she might have preferred a bath in the evening, her old pattern, replied:

> No, no. I've got quite accustomed to it now. And I get up early, about half past seven and I go into the kitchen … and get my breakfast. I just have coffee and toast. And then I take it back, with the paper, to bed and have it beside me and just stay there until Josie comes. Because you see it's no good me getting dressed. And that fits in very well, yes.

She had reordered her time and established a new morning ritual that was satisfactory and meaningful for her. Miss Henderson was similarly satisfied even though in her case the timing of the bath was sometimes unsure: 'I get up and play patience, and read my paper and have my coffee, and wait.' She did not mind sitting about in her night clothes.

> I mean it probably would be nice to have it um, a bit earlier than 12 o'clock, but I don't really grumble because I can still play patience or if I'm pushed, to write letters … I like pottering.

The sense of a new rhythm around care applied to the week also. Mrs Fitzgerald described how she structured her week around getting ready for the careworkers. 'Wednesday, which is today, she's been today – my big day, you see.' It had become 'the rose of my week'.

For these housebound recipients, help with bathing, far from coming at a 'meaningless' time, had itself become a source of meaning.

A bounded time

The interventions of domiciliary care are bounded by time as well as space. Just as home creates a special space for the operation of carework, so too do care visits define a special time, and the bounded nature of this time helps create the intimate space of bathing. It is a thing and a time apart. Stella describes the action of giving a bath in terms of the creation of a bounded space in which time stands still:

> Just peaceful it's kind of entering, it's like entering an inarticulate space and it's just like being there with somebody and sharing that intimacy and cutting through the chaos of every day it's like everything stops you know I mean because there is just a certain ritual pattern of how things have to be in order for a bath to be accomplished.

The domiciliary care visit creates a period of defined one-to-one contact. This is even more intense in the case of personal care where the worker is constantly in close, often physical, contact. In the case of housework, it is possible to some degree to ignore the person and just get on with the job. But help with personal care forces you to interact with and relate directly to them. Maintaining such human interaction, however, can be stressful for the worker. Some care recipients are depressing or boring to talk to. But the bounded time of the care encounter eases this. Careworkers are able to sustain contact with a deaf, slightly confused or grumpy person if it is only for a limited time. They can put their effort into relating, if they know it will not last for more than a prescribed period. The bounded time of the home care encounter is thus part of the sustainable intimacy of carework. This is in contrast to the way things operate in institutional care. There time is much more constant and homogeneous. Much of the time is surveillance time, and carework time flows on through twenty-four hours of the day. There are not the same defined periods of intensive time with a particular client. Rather, exposure to clients is constant. There is no beginning, no end, no escape. As a result careworkers tend to withdraw from interaction with clients and contact becomes homogenised, collective and distant.

Conclusion

The recipients of community care live their lives within a domestic world that is structured in terms of both time and space, indeed the two are interconnected, and we have seen how the spatial ordering of privacy and control has its parallel in the temporal ordering of domestic life. Care, in coming into this territory, brings its own rationalities, and these are in many ways in conflict within those of home and domestic life. The potential extent of such conflict can be seen in recent attempts to institute intensive care regimes at home, of which Hospital at Home schemes provide the strongest example, with bedrooms taken over by hospital equipment, halls cluttered by wheelchairs and oxygen cylinders, bathrooms turned into sluices, relatives driven back into siderooms, and twenty-four hour access to the house by staff the norm. Domestic time and space here become wholly subordinate to an institutional regime.

In general people in the study had not been made subject to anything like this degree. They retained considerable control over their homes and the domestic ordering of them. Home remained a buttress of self-identity and a significant source of power in the dynamics of the care encounter. The episodic nature of care, dipping and out of their lives, though sometimes a source of sadness, could also be a source of strength in that it meant that exposure to the world of service delivery and the demands of its rationality was limited. Domestic time and domestic space in large degree remained subject to their definitions.

5   The medical/social boundary and the rationalisation of community care

Baths in the community are predominantly provided by home care workers. This has not always been so. Up until the 1980s, personal care including bathing in Britain was regarded as a nursing activity, something that belonged to the medical rather than social care sector. The management of the body, at least in its naked or more vulnerable forms was seen as a nursing task, unless that body was contained within a formal care setting. During the 1990s, however, a series of changes, institutional, financial, political, produced a new configuration in which personal care came to be part of social care. As a result bathing is now fully integrated into the home care service. In this chapter we will explore the nature of these changes, in particular the impact of the reforms in the nineties that created the new community care. This has ushered in a more fragmented world of provision in which the private sector plays an increasingly significant role; and in the last part of the chapter we will reflect upon the nature of this market and in particular on features of the home care sector that pose problems for the application of economic rationality. Before doing so however we need to explore the meaning of the medical/social boundary, for it is the fact that bathing and personal care fall across this central faultline of community care that explains some tensions in its provision.

The medical/social boundary

Three features of this are of note. First, the boundary is constructed from the sedimentation of a number of divisions: institutional, financial, professional, ideological. Second, the relationship between the medical and the social is an unequal, asymmetrical one in which the medical represents the marked category and the social the unmarked. Third, the boundary is a shifting one; and where it falls has moved historically and across welfare systems. This movement and the fragmented, inexact nature of the boundary creates a zone of uncertainty, a grey area for provision and responsibility. This zone is differently conceptualised, but it encompasses such territory as 'long term care', 'social care', 'personal care'. The lives of older and disabled people, bathing and washing are frequently located in this frontier zone.

There is no single criterion that defines where the boundary between the medical and the social lies, for it is constructed from a series of overlapping divisions. Where the break in each of these falls can differ, so that the fault-line is ragged. The different layers, though conceptually separate rest on and reinforce each. Thus the high status that medicine enjoys as a knowledge system is linked to and gives ideological reinforcement to assumptions about the appropriate form of its funding.

In many ways the medical/social boundary is most defined and significant at the institutional level, in particular at the level of finance and payment. Across welfare systems there is a broad division between health care which is provided on a universal basis and free-at-the-point of use, and social care which falls into the means-tested territory where individuals are expected to fund themselves if they have the resources, and only rely on the state where they have not.

The exact pattern of provision is, of course, more varied than this broad picture allows. The account best fits tax-based universalistic systems like the UK and Sweden where health care is provided on a citizenship basis and broadly free at the point of use. Here health care is an unquestioned social right. It applies also to those countries like Germany and France with a social insurance model whereby health care is funded by compulsory insurance paid by employees and employers, and where an individual's contribution reflects income but benefits are standard (Wall 1996, Tester 1996). In these systems, coverage has been extended historically to the whole population – again underlining the special status of health care as a public good.

The major exception among affluent countries is the United States. Even here, however, the particular status of medical care is reflected in funding arrangements. Medicare does provide medical cover for all older people on a citizenship basis regardless of income, though it is compromised in terms of coverage – no prescription drugs – and by co-payments and deductibles. The coverage of Medicare thus itself reduplicates the status system within medicine, in that it broadly meets acute medical need but not chronic and long term care. American exceptionalism only really comes into play for those under pensionable age, where the responsibility for meeting health care costs falls to the individual, to be met either by personal resources or covered by private insurance or work place benefits. Those unable to meet these, face a pauperising test whereby they are required to spend down their assets in order to become eligible for the means-tested cover of Medicaid, which is a residual provision for the poor, covering both medical and social care costs.

If we turn to social care, it is clear that the sector is financially and institutionally more varied than is the case with medical care. Which forms of care are free and which charged for and at what rates varies across systems and has varied historically (Tester 1996, Glendinning *et al.* 1997, Royal Commission 1999). For example, home help in Sweden, the home of universalistic services, is charged for, but Swedish pensioners have high incomes. In both Britain and Denmark home care has been subject to a varying regimes, at some times free and at others charged for (Means and Smith 1985, Rostgaard and Fridberg 1998). In Germany home care has been drawn back across the payment boundary, and under the reforms of 1995 is funded not by individuals but collectively through the extension of the health care insurance to cover care at home. Previously such care was only available to individuals either by paying for it themselves or by seeking help from the means-tested social assistance system, a stigmatising procedure and one requiring the older person to have a very low income. In the US, the picture is complex and varies between the states. In general, home care is either funded by individuals themselves, or on a short term basis as an extension of Medicare (part of a strategy to reduce hospital costs), or on a means-tested basis by Medicaid as part of the long term care of the poor (Feldman *et al.* 1990, Benjamin 1993).

Broadly speaking, therefore, though there is variation, there is also a common pattern whereby social care is regarded as something that individuals should predominantly pay for themselves. It is regarded much like other day-to-day living or housing expenses – part of ordinary social life – and something therefore for which people are personally responsible, always with the proviso that those who cannot manage will be helped on a means-tested basis. The linking of social care to ordinary social life also appears to make it more subject to political judgements than is the case with medical care. This is reflected also in the variation in levels of home care across

Europe, suggesting that provision is more driven by policy choice than is the case with medical care (Royal Commission 1999).

The institutional division between health and social care is also reflected at the level of governance, in the sense of the level at which power is brokered and decisions made. There is a common pattern across western welfare systems whereby social care tends to be discussed, determined and often organised at the level of the municipality, whereas medical care is linked into the national level. This reflects a wider judgement about the nature of social care which has often been regarded as the responsibility of the local community and therefore more a matter for local option and control than is the case with health provision. This national focus also reflects the social power of doctors who are able to resist incorporation into the local state and locate themselves nearer the prestigious national level. This is particularly clear in the British case, where the medical profession in the 1940s and 1960s successfully fought off becoming subsumed under local authority control.

The fourth criterion of division is that of professional orientation. All health care professionals, however distinct their practice, in some sense look to medicine for their authority and knowledge base. It provides the integrating focus not just for the subordinated profession of nursing, but also for groups like radiographers, physiotherapists and occupational therapists: professions termed in a telling phrase, 'supplementary to medicine'. Social care activities by contrast fall under the professional remit of social work. Even though the majority of workers in the sector have no formal social work qualifications, their practice is shaped organisationally by social work values (though these are increasingly subject to challenge from managerialist approaches) and they work under senior staff who customarily have a social work qualification. The professional status of social work is, however, less strongly established (even within the profession itself) than is the case with medicine – that archetype of all that being a profession means – and social work's ideological control of the sector is less assured. It is the clash of these professional cultures of medicine and social work that causes many of the recurring problems in attempts at joint working across the divide. Social workers outposted to GP practices; multidisciplinary teams in mental health care; disputes between hospital consultants and field social workers on the issue of bed blocking: all provide examples of such institutionalised inter-professional conflict across the medical/social divide (Huntingdon 1981).

The division is not simply one of professional orientation but is rooted also in epistemology, in the sense of the differing knowledge-bases of the two sectors. As Estes and Binney note, the bio-medical model aligns itself with and is legitimated by its close association with science, the dominant and most powerful mode of thought in modern western society; and this endows it with an unquestioned authority (Estes and Binney 1989). Social care by contrast is rooted in the 'soft' social sciences or the – sometimes disputed – therapeutic tradition. It is not accorded the same status as the 'hard' knowledge of science. The division is also reflected in orientation to technology. Modern medicine is increasingly marked by high levels of technology, whether machine- or drug-based, and this is reflected within the status system of medicine itself, with high-tech, science-based interventions representing the prestigious heart lands of 'real medicine'. Social care by contrast rarely involves complex technology; and indeed the 'technological fix' tends to be poorly regarded, and is often seen as an evasion of the essentially social or interpersonal character of people's needs.

Medical practice is seen as involving skilled, physical interventions that act forcefully on the body and that could not be undertaken by another. Social care interventions by contrast are either more ethereal – counselling or other interpersonal work – or more mundane, providing day-to-day assistance of a practical sort. Dominant culture tends to deny the specialised character of the first and to downgrade the status of the second. In either case, they are seen as activities that most people could do without training, and the professional status of social care is thus undermined. At times, medicine deals with life threatening situations, and this dramatic quality endows it with additional importance. In certain situations, getting help can be literally vital. The social care professions rarely impact on people's lives in that way.

Of course, as epidemiological and social science research show, the wider social environment is far more significant than medicine in determining the pattern of life and death, longevity and suffering. At the level of social perception, however, medicine remains the more significant, and this feeds into the belief that medicine is 'necessary' and social care in some sense 'optional'. As we noted earlier in relation to payment and social rights, there a widespread acceptance that medical needs are 'real' needs and ones that at some level should be met by society. Indeed to define a problem as medical is to locate it in a policy discourse that is privileged. For example, showing that poverty makes people ill was contentious for a

Thatcherite government, as the furore surrounding the Black Report showed, because of the particular legitimacy that attaches to issues of health (Townsend and Davidson 1982). Simply referring to poverty and its miseries did not have the same political resonance.

These cleavages are not simply between the medical and the social, but are reduplicated within the territory of medicine itself. Nursing clearly belongs within the medical sphere; it is integral to the medical enterprise and it largely draws on the same bio-medical knowledge base. And yet, in many senses, nursing shares the same structural position in relation to medicine as does social work, carework or other forms of social care. The skills it emphasises as unique to the profession are ones that draw on a wider view of the patient encompassing him or her as an emotional and social being. Holistic traditions of nursing in particular aim to retain a sense of the person as an integrated being. Lawler (1997) argues that while medicine deals with the object body of science – anonymous, dependent, passive, reduced to the sum of its malfunctioning parts – nursing works to integrate the lived body of personal experience. Such accounts of nursing are of course highly idealised; and the reality of most modern nursing is one of time pressure, skill mix and fragmentation. However they do embody values that have affinities with those of the care sector more widely. At a more structural level, nursing suffers from even more acute problems in establishing its professional status and the independence of its knowledge base. The dominant account of the position of nursing remains one in which nurses are ancillary to doctors: there to carry out their orders and to provide the setting that makes their practice possible (Lawler 1991, Davies 1995).

These divisions are also gendered, both in the sense that the majority of nurses are female and that the tasks they perform and the qualities they exhibit are traditionally associated with women (Davies 1995). Nurturance, care, emotional labour, intimate bodywork are all conventionally regarded as female activities. Medicine by contrast rests on a set of 'masculine' values and practices in which scientific mastery, technological dominance and professional authority underwrite the status of the occupation even where, as is increasingly common, the tasks are performed by women. Gender thus operates not just at the level of the individual but, as Acker (1990) has argued, structures the nature of the organisation. This gendered division of labour is carried through into the caring professions more widely. The social work and social care sectors are predominantly staffed by women (Balloch *et al.*

1999), and the values they rest on – empathy, warmth, psychological discernment, practical, hands-on help – are once again those that are traditionally assigned to women.

The division between the medical and the social is also reduplicated in the distinction between cure and care. Both are properly part of medicine, and yet within the medical value system, cure has pre-eminence. Care *versus* cure also maps onto the division between acute and chronic care, which in turn relates to the medical/social boundary, in that with increase in pressure on resources, chronic care is increasingly re-categorised as social care.

These distinctions are played out in the ranking of medical specialisms. High-tech, science-based and cure-oriented specialisms have higher status compared with those with a large care component such as learning disability, rehabilitative medicine, psychiatry and geriatrics. The latter either manage chronic conditions or deploy skills that approximate to those of the ordinary social world, and as such approach the condition of social care. Such specialisms often attempt to take a more holistic view of the patient, and their practice is often undertaken in multi-disciplinary teams. They are also specialisms that are differentially staffed by women. From the perspective of the patient, these wider sympathies may be of value, but not from the viewpoint of medicine; and these are in general lowly regarded specialisms.

Lastly, setting is significant. The defining locus of modern medicine is the hospital. This was not always so historically. However with the rise of the infirmary in the nineteenth century and the development of drug-based, interventionist, modern medicine in the twentieth, the hospital has become the epi-centre of medical practice. It is where knowledge is generated, where the most complex work is undertaken and where the senior members of the profession are located. Community-based medical work does not enjoy the same status. In a similar way, it is ward-based hospital work that has defined the nature of nursing, and provides the source of status and legitimacy in the profession. Community nursing by contrast has always had a lesser, marginal quality to it, taking place 'out there', in territory that is not medical and that remains hidden from the hospital gaze. Community nursing has also traditionally been more concerned with the low status bed and bodywork of basic nursing care; until the 1980s this formed the mainstay of the work of district nurses.

As will have become clear, the relation between the medical and the social is not an equal one; and the two systems exist in an asymmetrical relationship in terms of status, power and political legitimacy. At a conceptual level, the medical is the defining sector and the social a residual category, representing 'all the rest'. Indeed the term 'the social' is itself problematic. It does not have the same coherence as the medical. In various of the divisions outlined above, other counter-terms, such as 'society', 'social work' and 'social science' are more appropriate, pointing up the unfocused nature of this side of the boundary.

In some senses it is better to think in terms of – not two systems – but one: that of medicine as a totalising system of knowledge and power that constructs all aspects of the social world (or those aspects it chooses to recognises) in its terms. This is the sense in which Foucault speaks of the medical gaze (Foucault 1973). By this account all aspects of life, the social world, personal relations, habits and feelings, are potentially relevant to the medical enterprise and capable of becoming subject to it. They form the background to medical practice and are admitted to the territory of medicine by the judgement of doctors as to their relevance. Medicine by this account is not so much a discrete territory in the social world, as a form of knowledge constituting aspects of it, in which the social is not a parallel or equal sphere but the setting in which medicine operates.

The dominance of the medical has not gone unchallenged. We have already noted the bodies of knowledge that have established the significance of social and cultural factors in the origin of health and illness. Since the 1960s, there has been a persistent critique of the medicalisation of life and the improper colonisation of sectors of it by the medical profession (Illich 1976). Within health and social care, the arguments have been most powerfully articulated within the disability movement, but they have been influential also in relation to learning disability, mental health problems, childbirth and terminal illness. In all these sectors attempts have been made to reassert the significance of ordinary social life and of models of care that draw on it (Oliver 1990, Brown and Smith 1992, Ward and Philpot 1995). With regard to older people, the debate has been less developed. This is partly because older people by virtue of their earlier lives are more strongly linked to the structures of ordinary life than is the case with people with learning difficulties or life-long disability, so that ordinary life models require less articulation. But it is also a product of agism and policy pessimism arising from the size of the planning population which means it is harder to debate and implement progressive approaches for this group.

As we have seen, the boundary between the medical and the social is not a fixed one, but shifting, subject to changing policy pressures. In recent years across welfare systems, there has been a marked tendency for the boundary to be drawn back and for more and more activities to be transferred across into the social care sector. Part of the reasons for this has been the desire to move away from medical dominance. Social care models are recognised as preferable, and

	Medical	*Social*
I Medical/social boundary		
Institutional/financial	healthcare institutions free at point of use	social care institutions responsibility of individual or means tested basis
	social right	residual right
Level of government	national	municipality
Professional orientation	medicine and professions ancillary to medicine	social work
Professional status	accepted	disputed
Knowledge base	bio-science	social science/therapeutics
	hard	soft
Application of technology	high and esteemed	low and not esteemed
Action	direct/bodily	diffuse/psychosocial
Legitimation and power	'real' life and death needs	more disputed 'needs'
	necessary	optional
II The boundary reduplicated within medicine		
	cure	care
	acute	chronic
	high status specialities	lower status specialities
	hospital	community
	ward	home
III A wider set of dichotomies		
	male	female
	father	mother
	doctor	nurse
	doctor	social worker
	rationality	emotion/nurturance
	cold	warm
	hard	soft
	public	private

supporting older and disabled people to live at home is widely endorsed as a policy. The main driver behind the transfer is however financial. Community care settings are perceived as cheaper than hospital: capital costs are lower (largely met by users), and low paid careworkers can be substituted for nursing staff.

The invention of the 'social bath'

Where does bathing care fall in all this? Bathing, as with other personal care, traditionally came under the remit of nursing, and in Britain in the post war era, baths were predominantly provided by the district nursing service. During the 1980s, however, under increasing pressure from hospital discharge and from the kinds of financial incentives described above, community nurses withdrew from this territory. They did this through the invention of the concept of the 'social bath'. This was defined negatively as the sort of bath that the community nursing service did *not* provide, because it was social rather than medical. In practice nearly all baths are 'social'. There are very few medical conditions that require a bath as such, and though extreme dirtiness may pose some health hazards, in reality the 'need' for a bath arises from social expectations and personal wishes. The significance of the term in the British debate derives from the fact that it allowed the nursing service to transfer a responsibility that had previously been accepted as falling under health over into social care. Managing the body is no longer of itself a nursing task.

The New Community Care and the restructuring of home care

The reforms of the 1990s, ushered in in Britain by the NHS and Community Care Act, were the product of a number of forces (Lewis and Glennerster 1996). The closure of the long stay hospitals, finally embarked upon in the 1980s after years of policy inaction, had implications for community care, and new forms of provision had to be built up. Government was keen to put a cap on the ever-expanding cost of residential care funded from the social security budget. There was a desire to end the 'perverse incentives' that arose from the failure to fund community care and that supported unnecessary institutionalisation. The proposed introduction of the internal market in the NHS encouraged the development of similar models in social care. The success of schemes based around case –

later care – management suggested that many older and disabled people could be supported at home at lower cost than in residential care (Davies and Challis 1986).

In relation to home care, the main drive for reform came from a sense that the service was failing to deliver the community care policy. Though the home help service had been the mainstay of domiciliary care from its inception in the post-war era (Dexter and Harbert 1983, Means and Smith 1985), it had remained limited in what it did and, in the view of many, poorly targeted (Social Services Inspectorate 1987). Mainly confined to housework, it did not by and large offer personal care. Provision was inflexible, mostly confined to the mornings and with no cover at weekends or in the evenings. The majority of allocations were for less than two hours a week, and intensive packages of care were rare. As a result authorities found it difficult to support more disabled people at home. Some authorities had developed flexible and innovative home care schemes, but they were limited geographically and often focused around a particular problem like hospital discharge (Ferlie *et al.*1989).

The form that the new arrangements took when they emerged in the 1990s was strongly influenced by the wider political climate and the impact of the New Public Management. This united a number of strands ideological, organisational, economic (Ferlie *et al.*1996). Two are of particular significance for home care. The first is the efficiency agenda with its use of market mechanisms and management techniques such as target setting and value for money audit. This was accompanied by a deregulation of the labour market, and the erosion of national pay agreements, together with a shift to new forms of corporate governance that mimicked those of the commercial sector. It was an agenda that had its roots in New Right thinking and a set of political assumptions about the relative inefficiency of public provision. The second strand derives from the impact of post-Fordist models of production. Fordist production rested on large, vertically-integrated structures; and large-scale corporations producing mass produced goods and public sector agencies delivering standard services are similar in their approach to production. In the post-Fordist world, however, the emphasis is on flexibility and speed of response, more individualised production and a shift from goods to services. Organisations have flatter structures and fewer staff. Management by hierarchy has shifted to management by contract, with a small strategic core linked to the larger periphery through relation of contact or agency.

The impact of these ideas can clearly be seen in the restructuring of social care as it emerged from the 1990s reforms in Britain. These introduced the purchaser/provider split requiring authorities to separate the functions of assessment and provision and to enter into agency relations with a number of local suppliers. In-house home care was increasingly hived off into a separate section, and exposed to the disciplines of the market. Some authorities privatised it altogether. Provision was no longer to be monolithic, but flexible and individual, and purchased in a social care market. Local authorities were given the responsibility of stimulating the independent sector. The labour market was de-regulated, and favourable local authority conditions abandoned.

In addition to these structural changes, there have been changes in what is provided. In the nineties, allocation shifted away from low levels of provision and towards more intensive packages. Between 1992 and 1996, the number of home care hours purchased increased by 50 per cent, but the number of individuals receiving help declined by 19 per cent. By 1996 the average allocation per week was 5.1 hours, representing a major process of intensification (Ford *et al.* 1998). Personal care is now fully integrated into the service (Balloch *et al.* 1999), and it is increasingly rare for home care to be allocated where no personal care is required. In areas like Coastville, a purely housework service funded by public money has ceased to exist. Older people who want help with housework and shopping now have to pay for it themselves or rely on voluntary sector provision. The retreat from the public provision of housework at a national level has been widely unpopular with both users and commentators (Walker and Warren 1996, Clark *et al.* 1998).

Community care in the 1990s was increasingly subject to charges. The post-war welfare legislation had empowered local authorities to charge for home help, but not all did and many remitted charges heavily where recipients were poor, so that by the 1970s, 71 per cent of recipients paid nothing (Dexter and Harbert 1983, Means and Smith 1985, Baldwin 1997). In the period from 1993, however, there was a rapid growth in the use of charges, and by 1995 an estimated 73 per cent of users made some contribution (Baldwin 1997, PSSRU 1998). This extended to individuals who were on income support. The cost of community care is thus increasingly borne by the users rather than the public purse.

The 1990s also saw the expansion of the independent sector. The size of the publicly-funded home care market is considerable, estimated at over a billion pounds a year in 1996. Laing and Buisson estimate that a further £420 million is spent on privately funded home care (Ford *et al.* 1998). The 1990 Act required local authorities to use 85 per cent of the social security transfer money to purchase care in the independent sector (Lewis and Glennerster 1996). Initially this was achieved largely in the form of residential care. During the nineties however the independent sector's share of local authority funded home care increased by more than ten fold: from 2.3 per cent in 1992 to 36 per cent in 1996 (Ford *et al.* 1998).

There continues to be considerable local variation in the pattern of purchasing, reflecting political views about the role of the private sector; as well as environmental factors such as dispersal of population that make it hard for the independent sector to operate in certain areas (Ford *et al.* 1998). In the study, Coastville had gone down the privatisation route early. Nearly all its provision was in the private sector, with only a rump of the old home care service remaining and that was increasingly required to operate according to commercial criteria. The London authority retained its in-house service, but was forced to buy in additional hours and staff from agencies; and there were plans for privatisation.

The rationalisation of home care

Home care, like the rest of the public sector, is increasingly conceptualised in terms of a business operation, and the growth of for-profit providers within the system has reinforced this. It is worth reflecting therefore on the nature of the home care sector and the potential for applying models of economic rationality to it.

Home care is a cottage industry. The independent sector in the UK is characterised by a large number of small, recently-established enterprises. Three-fifths of providers deliver services to less than a hundred clients, and only five per cent have more than five hundred clients (Ford *et al.* 1998). The barriers to entry are low, and in decaying coastal resorts like Coastville, new agencies spring up easily, undercutting more established firms. As a result the potential for consolidation or professionalisation of the sector is low. In the US, the emergence of state-wide contracting for Medicare in the eighties did allow for some consolidation of large scale for-profit chains where there were economies of scale in the contracting process and where regulatory expertise delivered financial advantage (Burbridge 1993). As yet, contracting in Britain remains small scale, and large chains can extract little competitive advantage. Indeed in parts of the country, contracting is largely spot contracting where arrangements are one-off and there are neither block or volume contracts (those being preserved for the in-house service). The profitability of the sector is low. As Burbridge comments in relation to the US, this is characteristic of public funding where third-party payers dominate the market and are able to use their oligopsonistic power to drive down prices to barely profitable levels (Burbridge 1993). It is certainly the case that local authorities in Britain have exerted heavy downward pressure on prices (Wistow *et al.* 1997). Typically agencies must fund their administration, recruitment, training and profit from a mark up of 25–30 per cent on the labour costs. A range of commentators have concluded that the nature of this market means that it is very difficult for agencies to maintain a stable workforce, provide decent pay or conditions of work or fund training; a conclusion echoed in the American literature (Feldman *et al.* 1990, Wistow *et al.* 1997, Laing and Saper 1999).

Wage levels in the private home care sector are low, well below the national average for female manual earnings (Ford *et al.* 1998). In many areas a dual labour market has developed with the local authority continuing to pay their in-house employees at a higher rates and with better terms and conditions. Private agencies typically pay a pound or so less per hour, provide no pensions, sickness or holiday pay, though changes arising from EU regulations have improved this situation. In so far as there have been 'efficiency gains' in the sector, they have been achieved through reducing the pay and conditions of workers. It is on their backs that the savings have been made.

Attempts to increase the efficiency of home care by other means has proved more difficult and this brings us up against certain recurring features of carework. It is, for example, difficult to accumulate demand, to save up care activities and provide them in concentrated and stable blocks (Feldman 1993). They have to be done when they are needed, and they follow their own, often body based, rhythms of time. Certain activities can be saved up, for example housework, and a weekly shop or clean up can cover activities usually done on a more frequent, often daily, basis. But personal care is not in general amenable to such consolidation. You cannot save up taking someone to the toilet, and then do it for two hours once a fortnight. This means that its provision is inevitably fragmented and expensive.

The one way in which efficiency gains can be made is by using institutional care. Gathering older people into one facility concentrates the work and allows for efficiencies of scale. It cuts out disrupted or travel time, and enables the bodies of older people to be marshalled and scheduled in an efficient way. It is one of the marks of institutional life for older people that their bodies become subject to these sorts of regulatory regimes in which they are fed, bathed, toileted according to schedule. One of the tensions in applying economic rationality to care comes from the link between efficiency and depersonalisation. As Goffman pointed out it is more efficient to allocate patients' coats from a collective pile than attempt to select and identify individual pieces of clothing. Diamond comments in relation to carework that simply 'strapping Juan into a diaper [rather than helping him to the toilet] was labour-saving, cost effective, time and motion efficient, profit accountable and documentable' (Diamond 1992: 180). The forces of rationalisation encourage such dehumanising practice. Making people subject to regimes of efficiency, of standardised responses, inevitably denies their individuality and humanity. In the queue for McDonalds this rationalisation of production matters little (Ritzer 1993), but in personal care it strikes at the heart of the quality of what is provided.

One of the classic ways in which productivity can be increased is by capitalisation, substituting capital for labour costs. In relation to bathing there is some scope for this in that there is a range of equipment on the market that enables people to get in and out of baths with greater ease. These fitments are expensive (in the order of a thousand pounds or more) and tend to be provided by individuals for themselves. Capital investment does not so much reduce staff costs, as enable the person to manage without help. In so far as it is an efficiency gain, it is so through the transfer of costs back into the private, informal sector. From the viewpoint of an agency, the efficiency gains are not sufficient to justify the investment in individual houses. There are too many sites of production. Furthermore, many bathrooms are extremely small and difficult to adapt. As a result, the bathing enterprise remains low tech, with minimal equipment and almost no significant capital investment, and it relies on the intensive use of low-paid workers.

Another area where there is scope for efficiency gains is in relation to rostering and rounds. What is required here however is consolidation in a locality such that demand becomes seamless, and unfunded hours in the form of travel time and spare units are minimised. This favours monopoly suppliers like the old home help service who were able to organise on a locality basis. Independent providers rarely achieve this and many are forced to operate across a wide geographical area picking up spot contracts. In this context, the alternative route to efficiency is through transferring the costs over to the workers. Thus careworkers in the independent sector typically have no guaranteed hours, work complex split shifts and are not paid for travel time; the cost of the slack is transferred to the worker.

The front line, intimate nature of carework can also pose problems for the application of commercial models. Care is by its nature interactive; it is something that is produced at the front line, in the houses and lives of individuals. As Baldock (1997, 1998) comments, production and consumption occur in parallel, and users and workers are co-producers of care. This makes it hard for organisations to control the production process. Unlike the factory, this is a form of production that is hidden and that takes place in territory that is private and not subject to the manufacturers' control. Carework, as Baldock notes, is marked by 'low compliance observability', remaining largely hidden from the gaze of manufacturers and funders. But how you are treated, the nature of the interaction, goes to the heart of what is provided. Commercial businesses in the service sector do attempt to control these interpersonal aspects, but this has been rare in relation to home care. Particular features of the sector suggest why this is so. Attention to managing and controlling the interface with customers is most characteristic of sectors like hotels or airlines where there is a strong possibility of customer exit. This has never been the case with home care. The low profit margins of the private sector and constrained budgets in the public means that there are few resources to invest in attempts to modify the behaviour of workers. There have been movements in the direction of training for home care workers, but financial pressure on agencies means that they are hard to fund. Rather this is a sector that had traditionally relied on naturalised concepts of good practice. Thus good home helps are so because they are naturally caring people. Careworkers can be relied upon to respond well to clients because of the sorts of people they are not because of any customer training they have gone through. This both reinforces the ideal of authenticity – they are nice because they *are* nice – at the same time as undercutting any claims that might be made for better pay or conditions on the basis of qualifications.

Conclusion

Though personal care is a key element in community care, for many years it was only provided on an uncertain, variable basis. Lying across the crucial fault line of the medical/social divide, it suffered from conflict around responsibilities and costs. The community nursing service perceived it as a marginal activity, to be fitted in after acute responsibilities had been met; and the old home help service saw body care as beyond the normal remit of their work. In the wake of the reforms of the 1990s, however, personal care has come to be fully integrated into social care, and it is now typically provided as part of the more complex packages of home care that have been the focus of the reforms. These shifts in provision have themselves created new gaps, notably in relation to lower levels of need in relation to housework and shopping. For those who do need personal care, however, the sources of help are now more clearly defined, even if still closely rationed.

Prominent among these sources are private sector agencies contracted to do the work via care management. Such contracts have brought a welcome element of flexibility into provision, though as we have seen, the nature of personal care is such that it poses difficulties for the full rationalisation of the sector. Profit margins are low and allow for little in the way of investment in the form of training or attempts to control and improve the front line of care which is left to naturalised concepts of good practice rooted in ideas about gender. Efficiency gains are difficult to achieve where contracting is local and small scale and where the potential for capitalisation is low.

Above all the close interpersonal nature of bodycare means that the principles of efficiency and of care are in conflict to a significant degree. Efficiency suggests that production should follow the model of McDonald's with an emphasis on repeatability, on efficiencies of scale, of standardised interactions and limited involvement (Ritzer 1993), but 'care' is structured differently. Care requires that the response be highly individual, specific to that person and to that moment. It is by its nature interactive, forged at the front line and cannot be separated from that setting or that interaction. Its remit is also unbounded, resting as it does on a response to the needs of the person as a whole rather than specific and localised care deficits. Care rests on an unbounded ethic that is in conflict with the focussed, instrumental nature of waged work, and we will explore this further in the following chapters.

6 The employment world of the careworker

Bates sums the sector up vividly:

> To the outsider, the 'caring' world may have appeared one of
> pink overalls, cleanliness, jangling keys, 'come along Annie',
> wheelchairs, walks around the grounds, trolleys, laundry, the
> ubiquitous institutional smell, dozing residents in television
> lounges. This was the re-presented, more acceptable face of the
> occupation, which in effect in terms of contemporary cultural
> constructs, was a 'heavy', 'dirty' job, steeped in taboo subject
> matter, such as the body, age, 'shit shovelling' and death. These
> social responsibilities were transported from the wider society to
> a sub-society, staffed largely by women. Within this sub-society, a
> partial and truncated version of 'caring' was enacted, involving
> constant tension between caring for and processing people.
>
> (Bates 1993: 20)

In this chapter we will explore the employment world of the front
line careworkers, looking at the labour markets that they find
themselves in and the contexts, both advantageous and difficult,
within which they work. This is in preparation for the following
chapters which discuss the central features of carework – as body
work and emotional labour. Carework is gendered work, but not
all workers are women, and in this chapter we will also address
the particular situation of male careworkers. Lastly, though this
book is about domiciliary care, many workers have experience of
residential care, and we will use their comments to explore some of
the structural factors that underlie differences between the two
sectors.

Who are these workers?

Home care is poorly paid but demanding work. Careworkers are predominantly drawn from working class women, though the pattern of employment also reflects the nature of local labour markets. In London the labour market for care is a fragmented one, in which employers compete for low paid staff against a relatively buoyant service sector. Inner London does not offer the large areas of working class housing that traditionally support a home care service, and most workers travelled in to the inner London borough from more distant and cheaper areas. The local authority in-house service had chronic problems over recruitment and retention, and was forced to rely heavily on agency staff. The for-profit and voluntary sector agencies drew on a similar pool of workers, though in addition they recruited strongly among transient workers: young, mostly white, women from countries like New Zealand, Zimbabwe, Australia, funding their travel in Europe by doing carework. In the racialised workforce of care, these young women are able to capitalise on their cultural capital as white and middle class. Such workers are also found in large numbers in the private, live-in sector, where the work provides accommodation as well as pay. The voluntary sector bathing service in the study, which was funded by the local authority but organised by a national charity, had a mixed group of staff that reflected the capacity of innovative schemes to recruit higher quality staff. A number of their careworkers – Sophie, Crystal, Jacqui – had degrees and many were transitional workers, doing bathing work on their way to something else, sometimes in the care sector, for example, graduate nursing or social work. They also recruited people working in the arts who were putting together work but the real focus of whose lives was elsewhere. One careworker was a dancer, another – Stella – a singer-songwriter. The London labour market is strongly racialised and a large proportion of the London careworkers were black. In addition there was evidence of an earlier racialisation, in that many of the older white women workers were Irish.

Coastville is a deprived area with high unemployment, and care-work was one of the few sectors offering jobs. The profile of workers in Coastville was nearer the classic picture of home care. The majority of staff were women of middle years fitting work around children, though there were also a proportion of younger women. However, just as their employment was now more fragmentary than under the old home help service, so too did their lives appear to be. A number were single parents, some had disabled partners or children, and many were piecing together work as they could. In Coastville the workforce was almost entirely white.

What else might they be doing? Apart from the group for whom carework was a transition to other more highly paid work, the majority of careworkers in the study faced limited employment choices. Some had worked in different, but also low paid, sectors like retail, factory or field work, but the majority had come to carework either direct or via carework in institutions. With few or no qualifications they faced a constrained set of options in the employment market. For some, carework as a positive choice; factory or office work was boring and unsatisfying and offered none of the interpersonal rewards of care. For others, it was simply something that they could do and that was available locally. For a small group of older white women in London, carework appeared to have been a forced option, other more attractive sectors such as office or retail work being closed to them because they were approaching or over retirement age. Among the black careworkers, though many were positive about their work, there was a sense that their employment options were additionally constrained. The labour market is racially segregated, and the more middle-class and genteel unskilled work, like being a receptionist or working in a shop, tends to be differentially occupied by white women, leaving heavier, messier and less attractive occupations in catering and care for black workers.

The attractions and disadvantages of carework

In employment terms, carework is disregarded, bottom of the heap work. Bates (1993) and Skeggs (1997) note that caring courses are the least regarded of training options, and they present the work as something that young women with few qualifications or choices in the labour market learn to adjust their horizons to accept. Skeggs, in her analysis of class and gender formation among young women, argues that choosing carework and developing a self identity as a caring person is a response to situations where employment prospects are bleak, sources of self esteem few and cultural capital in the sense used by Bourdieu low. Carework offers a chance to deploy what little cultural capital that they have in the form of gender identity. Bates argues that carework is reasonably accessible to such young women by virtue of their cultural preparation in the working class family. The quality that the courses and the jobs were looking for was a certain toughness in dealing with the unpleasant aspects of the work, but one constrained by gender socialisation from developing into violence: employers wanted women who had learnt to rein in their reactions. The classes were most successful with girls from the rougher sections of the working class, and Bates argues that class-gendered cultural preparation in the family was crucial in explaining the successful adjustment of trainees to the work.

Careworkers are aware that surrounding society does not have a high opinion of their work. Bates describes how young women on the courses kept quiet about their activities, recognising a slight revulsion among their friends at what the work entailed. Part of this, as we shall see, relates to its character as 'dirty work'. Bartoldus and her colleagues in the United States similarly reported that 'workers said that they believed that the general public viewed them as "unskilled maids" who did society's "dirty work" '. They saw perceptions of their jobs as similar to attitudes towards housewives: "Nobody respects a housewife that much ... it's not a real job" '(Bartoldus *et al.* 1989: 207).

At times careworkers were angry at the denigration of their work. One manager described how one of her staff had gone for a college interview and was asked "What on earth is someone like you doing that kind of work for, you're bright, intelligent, educated'. The worker felt angry and belittled; she was 'equating me with someone sweeping the streets ... Sort of the lowest of the low'. Some workers consciously resisted the low esteem in which carework is held and asserted instead the intrinsic value of the work and the interpersonal rewards that it could offer. From their perspective, it is important work: 'It's lack of knowledge really that they think it's a lowly job, but it's just lack of knowledge on their part.'

Despite the low status, careworkers are in general very positive about their work. Feldman and her colleagues (1990) found that American home care aides, despite the otherwise harsher context for their work, also expressed high overall satisfaction. The NISW study of the social services workforce found that home helps had higher levels of satisfaction in relation to nearly all aspects of their work than social workers, managers or residential staff (Balloch *et al.* 1999). The finding is striking because jobs at the bottom of the organisation are in general associated with higher stress and poorer morale. The key lies in the direct nature of the interpersonal rewards, and the freedom from close control.

Home care is usual for a low level job in its relative absence of direct supervision. Workers are out in the community and not under the thumb of a manager. 'I like to be my own boss really,' explained one. Freedom from being controlled and reprimanded was important. 'Being able to chat and not get told off,' added another. 'In a client's home, you're your own boss anyway. You just go in and get on with it and if you think you've done wrong then you know what to do.' Span of control is recognised as a key variable determining morale at work; and careworkers are able to control the pattern and pace of their work. The job entails variety, and the workers move around the locality relatively freely, fitting in their own shopping or phone calls, popping back to do things at home. In London, the work offered in addition the chance to wander around an attractive and fashionable district. This sense of space and of self direction was significant for morale. Domiciliary carework appeals to people who are relatively independent. For nurses, community work has always provided an escape route for those who find hospital life claustrophobic, or are resistant to the close control of managers and doctors. Home care managers recognise that domiciliary work requires staff who enjoy and are able to work independently, and in their view, the extra responsibility justifies the slightly higher rates that are paid. (Interestingly in the US, the pattern is reversed and home care workers are paid significantly less than those who work in nursing homes (Feldman *et al.* 1990).)

Home care work as we have seen is increasingly provided in fragmented and flexible forms. This cuts both ways for workers. For some, it can be attractive, allowing them to pursue personal projects like Stella's songwriting. For one or two, this fragmented work allowed them to combine paid work with family obligations, popping back to visit a disabled child or elderly mother, and evening work sometimes fitted well with a working partner who could look after children. But the fragmentation was also one of the least attractive parts of the work. Split shifts left workers with awkward time on their hands, and meant that the working day stretched out to cover all waking hours. Evening work could also have its dangers. One careworker in Coastville described a nasty incident when: 'I did have a run in. This car stopped with a load of blokes in and one got out and I just legged it down the road and I was so trashed I wouldn't go in the next night.' Though she had been badly frightened, she could not afford to give up the work.

Among some of the older workers there were also anxieties about health. Dawn, a woman in her fifties, who had recently had a bladder operation and had arthritis, was frightened that her knee might give way when supporting a client. Staff face the common dilemma of manual workers as they grow older, of recognising that they are not as strong or robust as before, realising it is increasingly easy to injure themselves, and yet having no option but to do the work. Clients could also be violent. By and large in the study this was not so, as violence is associated with dementia which is also associated with institutionalisation; for workers in residential care, however, it can be a major source of injury.

Lastly many careworkers faced material difficulties in accomplishing their work. Conditions in people's homes can be problematic: dirty, damp, cramped. Bathrooms were often tiny. The equipment that was meant to be there, rarely was, or the space did not allow it to be used properly. This meant that the strict rules about manual handling promulgated by the agencies were often impossible to follow. As Desiree explained, manual handling rules were: 'a load of rubbish, because we're still lifting ... We've been shown all these gadgets at this manual handling course. I've never seen any of them (laughing).'

The male careworkers

So far we have treated careworkers as if they were women, but men also work in this sector, and a number of the agencies had one or two men on their books (though some of the smaller ones had none). In Coastville home care the ratio was seventy-two to four. Carework is commonly perceived as women's work and it is interesting therefore to ask how far and in what ways the experiences of men are different.

All the male interviewees had in some sense drifted into the work, and none had chosen it as a career. Geoff, for example, having left school at 16, had gone into the army, done clerical work and then trained as a carpenter, but finding opportunities were few in Coastville, had taken up carework. Barry in London, having failed to get a job after an HND in leisure studies, looked at a range of low-level jobs in shops, stores and offices; home care work was the first thing that had come up. Joshua had come from Sierra Leone hoping to train as an accountant, but he had no money to study and found maths difficult. He got night work in the kitchens of a newspaper and then, answering an advert for a bathing attendant, used that day job to piece together a wage.

In many ways the context of their employment was very similar to that of the women: fragmented career paths and limited opportunities in which work had to be pieced together. The contrast lay in the way that the gender order, which 'naturally' led women into these areas of work, operated in reverse for men. Carework was not an obvious occupation for a man. Joshua took up the work by chance (though he also had a girlfriend who was a home help) but was now considering training as a psychiatric nurse. All three men had discovered an ability and liking for the work in the context of limited options, and in doing so had overridden traditional gender stereotypes. But in Barry and Geoff's cases, a certain defensiveness remained in their accounts. Carework is women's work, and for them this implicitly raised issues of sexuality and status.

It is important to stress that the central experiences of carework were similar for men and women. They valued the same aspects – the emotional reward of helping, the warmth of interpersonal exchanges, and the freedom and autonomy of the job – and they experienced the same problems – the emotional strain of the work and the need to set limits on personal involvement. The rewards and tensions of the work, although often associated with the particular character of women and gendered identities, are an inherent part of the job. This is not to deny that carework is gendered work, for the job is indeed structured around assumptions about women, but it is the job that is gendered and this can be at odds with the gender of the person who occupies it.

There was some evidence that male workers approached aspects of the job, particularly the negotiation of intimate care, in a different way. Janet Shannon, the manager of a not-for-profit agency, felt that men were consciously professional and efficient in manner whereas women used jokes and informality:

> Most males are fairly professional when they enter someone's home to deliver personal care. They have a professional approach because they're gonna get a difficult task done and I think to adopt this terribly professional approach. [Women] joke and they laugh and they sort of make all sorts of silly comments ... because this difficult thing has to be done or embarrassing bit has to be done. Whereas I think males are far more likely to take this clear professional approach.

In all cases in the study male careworkers were confined to male clients. Geoff would have been happy to assist women and he had done so in residential homes. He felt it made no difference:

> If somebody said to me 'This woman doesn't mind you going in and giving her a wash, do you mind?' I'd say 'No', 'cos to me I'm just going in and giving them a wash. That's it. It's just like washing a man, just go in, look at them – just look at them as a

person, not a sex – and that is it, over and done with.... I had to take women to the toilet, change their pants. Get them up when they were wet, change their clothes, get them dressed but then homes like that have different rules to what [Coastville social services] do.

But he was aware that home care was different and that practices that were acceptable or tolerated in residential homes were not in a domestic setting where 'accusations can fly, not from my part, but from the woman's side'. It is clear that setting was significant here. A male careworker going into a female client's home was perceived as problematic. This was partly because the interchange would be more hidden than in an institutional setting, but it also reflected deeply felt ideas about intimacy and space. Interchanges in a private home have a different quality to them; they are by their nature more intimate. Concern about male careworkers also reflects more general anxieties about males in the care sector. The exposure of the extent of sexual abuse of children and vulnerable adults in care homes has resulted in a situation where all male workers are to some degree under suspicion. Male careworkers have to careful and this reinforces a 'professional' approach.

All three men were aware of an undercurrent around the issue of their sexuality. They were all heterosexual, but men who work in caring occupations suffer from a series of cultural assumptions that since this is women's work, men who do it must be effeminate and therefore gay (assumptions also reported by Warren 1994). They also suffer from the homophobia of male clients, or at least from male anxieties about intimate tending by another man. Hegemonic masculinity in the west is closely constructed around the rejection of the homosexual (Connell 1995). Men share ideas of other men as sexually predatory, and assuring oneself that the careworker is not a homosexual was important for some clients.

The male careworkers were more ambitious. Though they all valued carework, two of them were also clear that if any internal opportunities for advancement arose they would take them, and both had already moved across to work in the office part time. As Barry explained: 'that's what I intend to do, just go up, up the ladder'. In this they were following a pattern characteristic of males in female-dominated occupations, whether nursing, social work or teaching, whereby men take all opportunities they can get for advancement, even though this takes them away from the core activities of the work. Women remain more committed to this core and, for a variety of reasons, reluctant to take the managerial route. For men, female dominated professions offer easier advancement, but lower status.

As Williams (1989) argues in her study of men and women in non-traditional gender occupations (male nurses and women in the military), there is a fundamental asymmetry in the economic consequences of gender maintenance for men and women that works to the benefit of men. In the army men dominate the institution and are able to deny women full participation, particularly in the key role of combat, thus segregating them into low status peripheral areas. Women in the military pose a threat to men that is deeper than just their jobs. Men's masculinity is threatened by the presence of women able to do jobs previously reserved for masculine men. In relation to nursing, though men have sometimes been subject to exclusionary practices (for example midwifery), these do not normally halt their progress. Rather the differential treatment of men and women benefits men in nursing, giving them greater prestige and authority. There is however a certain stigma involved in doing women's work, and the stereotype of gayness is part of the penalty men pay. Nursing work, Williams argues, is also work that is deemed below or demeaning for men, and this aspect is closely linked to its bodily character, particularly the bedpan and shit cleaning aspects. As a result, men are encouraged and enabled to take the route out of such activity. The glass escalator takes them up and away. In carework this process is compounded by concerns about sexual abuse. Authorities look askance at men who linger too long at the front line of care.

The gendered character of the work is also closely linked to status. Barry was particularly conscious of this, caught in the tension between the rewards and responsibilities of the work and its low status in the eyes of the wider world. He felt that the work was valuable and worthwhile, and other jobs he might do were less interesting, but at the same time resented its poor public esteem: 'Carework. I say it's undervalued ... isn't necessarily any less worthy than the other things.... It is really a difficult job, but classed as a sort of low skill job, a manual job.'

This concern with status marked him apart from the female respondents and reflected expectations he and others held about what work men should aspire to. He was clear that the status of carework was below the norm for men: 'Why become a carer if you're a fella ... why *aspire* to that job?' He saw carework as a dead end job and had moved across into supervisory work in the office 'for my own sort of self-esteem, or for my own sort of self-worth, it's necessary to have that sort of sense of development.'

Struggles around self esteem and status emerged particularly strongly in his account of competitive relations with male clients who had in their past lives been powerful and dominant figures. Hegemonic masculinity, as Connell (1995) argues, is not necessarily to the advantage of all men; and it needs to be seen as the means whereby select groups of men create and sustain positions of power against other men as well as women. We will return to the ways in which gender and class intersect in the last chapter.

In many ways the experience of carework is similar for men and women: the nature of the work, the character of the labour market. But this experience is mediated through different expectations about gender that put limits on what men may do, and reduce their status in their own eyes and those of the wider world. But in doing so they also point men in directions that are to their long-term advantage.

Institutional contrast

Carework is a generic term, encompassing a set of tasks that is common to hospital, residential and home care. But the setting in which the tasks are performed significantly affects their character. In this section we will look at a rival site of care in the form of the residential home, using the comments of careworkers to explore the different dynamics of the two social spaces.

The literature on residential carework has a much harsher tone than that on home care, and the social world it describes is grimmer and colder. Partly this may result from the use of participant observation that allows for a franker and less mediated account. But it also seems to reflect a reality. Many of the careworkers in the study had worked in both sectors and they were clear that they did not want to return to residential work. They perceived the regimes as harsh and uncaring, and felt that the staff were cold and sometimes nasty. Lee-Treweek (1996, 1998) describes how residential workers relished the toughness that was required to do the work and regarded careworkers who worked in other, softer sectors with some contempt. Barry commented: 'you get some horrible ones.... they're not so caring in a home, I've got to be honest.' Judy, the home care manager in Coastville, agreed that residential staff were different, harder, 'more militant', less willing to internalise the ethic of caring.

The conditions of work in residential care are also less attractive. Levels of control are high and you are constantly under the thumb of the manager. As Terri commented: 'At least when you're out in the community you haven't got someone constantly looking over your shoulder, telling you exactly how you should clean the toilet.' The work was claustrophobic and repetitive. Barry: 'You start at eight and you finish at five and you're just in one place all the time ... you're always doing the same thing every day, every day.' There was none of the variety or freedom of domiciliary work.

The pace of work was also harder, with enervating levels of heat and constant activity. One worker said 'I was so tired I used to go to bed at eight o'clock at night.' Most respondents had worked in small private residential homes where owners operated on narrow margins and drove the staff hard. Staff felt that as a result of this pressure of work they: 'couldn't give the care that you were expected to give ... if there's only three of you to do 47 people, there's no way you can give the care that you know you should be giving.' They never spoke to residents: 'You can't sit and talk to them, you don't have time. So it's sort of rushing all the time and you haven't got time to spend the time of day with them.'

Judy agreed that the regimes were different, and she summed up a number of crucial features of this:

> When you're actually in a client's home, that client is actually more dependent on you. You're more in a one-to-one with that client. When you're actually in a residential you don't have to be – the interaction isn't there so much, because there's other staff about. And if they're walking down a corridor, they'll walk past a client without saying good morning or anything like that, whereas if you're actually in a client's home, and it's in the morning, you speak to that client. So I do think the attitudes are different, the mentality is different.

Institutional work involves constant exposure to residents. Time in care homes is unremitting; it stretches out without limit, enduring through the whole twenty-four hours. Workers cannot escape from contact with residents. By contrast, one of the characteristics of higher status workers like doctors or social workers, is that they can limit their exposure to clients. They do not have to deal with them over long periods of time. This makes possible, in theory at least, direct engagement. Residential careworkers however like ward staff have to remain in the company of the mad, sick or confused hour after hour, day after day. Such exposure is hard to endure, and makes it almost impossible to sustain real engagement. Workers defend themselves by withdrawal, by developing a certain air of brisk distance, by letting their gaze slide over the heads of the residents. As

Judy said: 'If they're walking down a corridor, they'll walk past a client without saying good morning.' At best this militates against the real engagement that is at the heart of caring; at worst it provides the foundation for abuse, in that abuse thrives where the personhood of the individual is denied.

Residential care is batch living, in which the pressure of numbers means that individuals are treated as one of a group. There are efficiency gains in managing people collectively. One member of staff can watch a lounge full of residents. But batch living is the negation of the self. It is difficult to maintain a sense of identity where space is largely collective, privacy has limited meaning and residents have few possessions with which to maintain their sense of self.

Staff in care homes rarely work alone, but are usually part of a group of workers among whom a certain solidarity builds up. Workers regard the care home as their territory, and residents are under their control and management. Their tasks are to maintain order against the endless entropy of leaking bodies and frail limbs. It is a constant process of fire fighting, in which the bodies of residents have to be cleaned, managed, and arranged. Workers look to their colleagues for help with this. As a result, a dynamic builds up in which it is careworkers against the residents. Workers often withdraw to the office or kitchen – space that is out of bounds for residents – to chat among themselves, keeping an eye out through the door for trouble. They talk over the heads of residents. It is inevitable that they should find their colleagues more attractive sources of conversation than residents: they do not suffer from problems of deafness or confusion and above all, they are like them, they share the same interests, the same work conditions. People always prefer to socialise with those who are like themselves. There is an inevitable camaraderie around the workplace that excludes the residents.

Domiciliary care is different on all three particulars. As we have seen, it takes place in space that belongs to the client and that is saturated with reminders of their identity and past. Often the space is still controlled in such a way as to deny the dominance of the worker, and the structural pattern of privacy is maintained. Careworkers' exposure to clients is also time limited. They come for an hour or so, but then they go, and this makes possible one-to-one contact. However difficult or trying the person is, there is natural point of closure. This contrasts with the residential home, where exposure can only be limited by psychic withdrawal. For the client too, the time is not continuous, but defined and structured. The worker comes and the worker goes, leaving the home to reassert itself. It may be a reassertion of loneliness, but it is a reassertion of space and time that is theirs.

Lastly, careworkers in the domiciliary sector by and large work alone. This once again supports contact on a direct one-to-one basis. For that defined hour or twenty minutes giving a bath, they are wholly in the presence of the client, and there are none of the rival attractions of the work group. The client may be hard to follow or a little confused, but there is no one else to talk to. The dynamics of the situation support human interaction, whereas those of the residential home deny it. Mrs Colegate, a women with MS, recognised this dynamic when she got to the point when she needed two workers to help her, and she was concerned that they would talk over her. At first this did happen but:

> I thought well, I can't have this, talked about their personal problems and that, I thought they're not here for that really they're here for looking after me so I joined in and now they talk to me as well you see ... otherwise you get left out.

She had the confidence to assert herself and to prevent the workers withdrawing into their own interests over her head, but then she was in her own home.

Conclusion

Domiciliary carework is not well rewarded in terms of either money or status and most of the staff who work in this area do so in the context of limited employment options. But the work itself, although at times difficult or stressful, brings its own rewards. Indeed few jobs contain such directly positive feedback. Seeing the pleasure your company and help bring, knowing that you are needed and valued, are important sources of self esteem for staff whose rewards in the formal world of work are otherwise not likely to be great. The terms under which the work is performed are also better than might at first appear. Domiciliary carework, for all that it is poorly paid and often fragmented work, does allow for a certain amount of freedom and control. Above all workers are not directly under the thumb of supervisors, something unusual in low level work, and this fact is clearly reflected in their high levels of morale. Domiciliary carework is also free of many of the tensions of institutional care. Workers who worked in the community had by and large chosen to do so, and they had rejected the regimes of residential care that many of them had experienced. So despite the limited options that these workers face in the labour market, many had exercised a positive choice in working in this area, and they felt that the work that they did was valuable in its own right.

This was as true for the men as the women. The key difference lay however in the future prospects of the two groups. Male careworkers were much more likely to pursue opportunities that took them away from the core activities of care. In this they are helped by gendered assumptions about what sorts of work are appropriate for men. Rather than excluding them from care in a negative way, these assumptions operate to encourage men to take the path of advancement that takes them away from the front line of care, and will be to their long-term advantage.

7 Carework as bodywork

Carework has traditionally been presented in ways that downplay its character as bodywork. In this chapter we will explore the nature of bodywork, focusing on how careworkers manage and interpret these aspects. One of the reasons why the bodywork element in care has been neglected is that it deals directly with the negativities of the body, the aspects of unboundedness that modern culture is reluctant to address (Lawton 1998). Careworkers manage these aspects on behalf of wider society, and we will explore some of the techniques that they use to do this, in particular the ways in which they put limits on the physical intimacy of the work. Before doing so, however, we need to address the nature of bodywork more generally.

Bodywork

Bodywork involves working directly on the bodies of others. (I am excluding here the 'work' that individuals undertake on their own bodies.) Typically it involves touching, manipulating and assessing the bodies of others, which thus become the objects of the worker's labour. The aim of such interventions can be medical, therapeutic, pleasurable, aesthetic, erotic, hygienic, symbolic; and it encompasses a range of practitioners: doctors, nurses, careworkers, alternative practitioners, hairdressers, beauticians, masseurs, sex workers, undertakers. The contexts in which they work are very varied. However, there are certain common themes in the work, and in the account that follows I will draw out those relevant to the construction of carework.

The most obvious parallels are in the health care sector. Though medicine deals with the body, it does so in a particular and circumscribed way, constructing it in terms of the object body of science, distant, depersonalised (Lawler 1997). Direct bodywork is not central to the activity of doctors, indeed medical practice is constructed in such a way as to limit such involvement; and professional status is marked out in terms of distance from the body. We can see this in the history of the medical profession, in which the elite London-based physicians of the seventeenth and eighteenth centuries rarely if ever touched their patients but practised their art by eye and by nose, leaving direct hands-on work to lesser status bonesetters and apothecaries, or the barber-surgeons. It was only the coming of modern medicine, with its asepsis, anaesthesia and high-tech focus, that allowed surgery to be reassigned to an elite, virtuosi status; though even here it retained a certain grossness in its associations, as illustrated in the symbolic representation of the bodies of doctors whereby physicians were presented as lean and cerebral, and surgeons stout and vulgar as befitted the crude physicality of their work (Lawrence 1998). Much of the ritual and drama of the ward round centres on protecting doctors from the loss of status involved in bodily contact. Distancing techniques like white coats, bodily stance, arrival and departure are typical of how such high-status workers deal with the body element in their work. Doctors perform relatively little direct bodywork and where they do it is largely confined to the high-status activity of diagnosis or mediated by high-tech machines. Where it is part of treatment, it is usually delivered by lesser practitioners like physiotherapists or nurses.

Nursing ironically shares many of these the ambivalences. Though bodywork is at the heart of nursing, it has an uncertain status. Nursing is organised hierarchically, so that as staff progress, they move away from the basic bodywork of bedpans and sponge baths towards high-tech, skilled interventions; progressing from dirty work on bodies to clean work on machines. Despite the attraction of holistic approaches (in the academy at least), in recent years this traditional hierarchy has been reinforced by the introduction of skillmix in which basic bed and bodywork is confined to the lowest skill, one which may not indeed require a trained nurse. This dematerialising, aetherialising tendency has been noted by a number of commentators (Dunlop 1986, Littlewoood 1991, Savage 1995, Davies 1995), and Dunlop argues that the recent emphasis on psychological dimensions of the patient and indeed the whole educational project with its tendency to academicise nursing, represents a further flight from the bodily in pursuit of higher status forms of knowledge and practice. The highest status work in nursing – research, management, education – involves no bodies at all.

The bodywork element in nursing is sometimes interpreted in terms of the symbolically charged character of the nurse's own body (Wolf 1988, Littlewood 1991, Bashford 2000). Nurses in their management of the body and its wastes are able to move across the boundaries of the sacred and profane acting as a mediator of pollution. The symbolic purity of the nurse, it is argued, means that she is able to deal with the discordant, 'dirty' aspects of the patient without losing status. There is however also a counter symbolism in which the bodies of nurses are themselves sexualised by virtue of their familiarity with the body in general; and nurses commonly feature in popular stereotypes and male fantasies.

The second main sector of bodywork centres on trades that aim to beautify the body: hairdressers, beauticians, manicurists (Gimlin 1996, Sharma and Black 1999). The sector is biased towards women since they have traditionally been more concerned with – or required to present – a groomed and beautified body, but it encompasses men also, with barbers and hairdressers. Improving appearance is the central aim, but themes like pleasure are also important, and beauty trades are also body pampering trades, encompassing massage, aromatherapy and other sources of sensuous enjoyment. Again there is a gendered element. Women are permitted by wider culture to enjoy such interventions; tending, grooming, touching are accepted as a natural and appropriate; though for men, as we shall see, their meaning is more ambivalent, bordering on the territory of prostitution.

Many of these interventions are packaged in the language of therapy – beauty 'treatments'. This brings us to a third focus, which is alternative medicine, for the boundary between beauty and health treatments is a highly permeable one. Alternative medicine in its pursuit of what Sharma and Black (1999) term 'deep health' aims to integrate the lived body with the mind or spirit. Bodywork is a prominent feature of alternative therapies, many of which, like osteopathy, chiropractice, massage, involve direct hands-on contact. Bodywork is also prominent in self-therapies like Alexander technique, yoga, pilates. Alternative medicine draws heavily on touch both in diagnosis and treatment. The healing power of touch is central to many therapies, and lies at the core of the association of holism, spirituality and healing in this tradition. A personal relationship with the practitioner is also part of the tradition. For many users, such treatments are an alternative or complement to orthodox medicine in the context of chronic illness or conditions like cancer. But for a significant number, they are part of the pursuit of a wider concept of wellbeing that echoes other preoccupations of the body in post-modernity. Wolkowitz (1998) sees such trades as exemplifying the 'new bodywork', in which recreation and therapy are linked. Here work on the body is non invasive, confined to the surface, largely pleasurable and freely sought by clients, often in a market place of freelance practitioners. This she contrasts with the orthodox medical sector, where touch is rarely therapeutic in itself and where contact may be painful and invasive.

But bodywork also borders on the more ambivalent territory of sexuality; and lurking in the wings of any discussion of bodywork is the question of prostitution. Much bodywork consciously attempts to bracket off the realm of desire and assert the neutral asexual character of its interventions. Just as Naturism emphasised its non-sexual character, so bodywork therapies, even those that value sensuousness and pleasure in the body, present their activities – such as massage – as non-sexual. Prostitution is one of the oldest forms of bodywork, recurringly associated with the bath house, the beauty trades, the massage parlour; as well as, in male fantasy, with that other area of bodywork – nursing. Prostitution is a stigmatised form of work that centres on servicing the desires of a dominant customer. Though it has at times been treated as a form of immorality (where the immoral act is to engage in relationships outside the prescribed limits of marriage and directly for money), what is low about the work is that it involves body servicing in a directly subordinated way in relation to sex. This may involve contact like massage that mimics other forms of bodywork, or it may involve directly using your own body or allowing it to be used. Either way the worker is subordinated in a directly bodily way to the desires of the customer. The question of subordination is at the heart of many of the tensions around bodywork, and the phrase 'body servant' captures something of this. It is that role that workers seek to avoid, and that professionals above all resist. Subordination when it centres on the body takes on a particularly intimate and personal character. Who directs whom becomes all the more highly charged when the site of struggle is the body. It is because of this that the power dynamics of bodywork can tip either way – into the demeaned territory of the prostitute, or the dominant and controlling creator of docile bodies.

Finally bodywork can also involve the less attractive aspects of the body. Occupations that deal directly with the body and its wastes are recurringly regarded as low in status, on the border of the polluted. In caste societies, sweepers and barbers are drawn from low castes or untouchables. In modern western societies, such jobs are done by the lowest paid, least regarded workers; being a lavatory cleaner epitomises a low status job, however much people recognise that it needs to be done. Dealing with dead bodies involves similar ambivalences. Undertakers in western society often find they are avoided socially; and they are traditionally a self-recruiting, family-based group. Strong taboos adhere in their work; and their role is to process death and decay in such a way that its bodily character is hidden.

To sum up, bodywork is highly ambivalent work. At times it verges on area of taboo in connection with sexuality or human waste. It is potentially demeaning work, and when undertaken by high status individuals it is typically accompanied by distancing techniques. There is a recurrent dematerialising tendency whereby status in a profession is marked by distance from the bodily. At the same time, bodywork is closely linked with pleasure and emotional intimacy. Therapies and techniques that rest on it create a zone of physical enjoyment and wellbeing. Body work is also gendered work, differentially performed and received by women. Lastly, aspects of subordination and domination are of central significance, and can create an unstable, ambiguous quality to its social exchanges.

The silenced nature of bodywork

Bodywork lies on the borders of the taboo. All cultures have patterns of belief and practice which govern and proscribe behaviour relating to the body. In the west, our way of dealing with the body, sexuality and dirt is to take them into a privatised context that makes them relatively inaccessible to us as a subject for social enquiry (Lawler 1991). There is little or no public discourse of the body and its functioning. It is rarely referred to directly, beyond the world of childhood, intense intimacy or crude jokes. This chimes with the form of analysis presented by Elias (1978).The body occupies a territory where language itself is problematic, awkwardly polarised between the medical-clinical and the vulgar-demotic. Lawler (1991) notes how nursing texts are coy about what the basic work of nursing entails. It is regarded as 'obvious', and the actual embodied reality, either glossed over or fragmented into a series of what are termed 'personal care deficits'. In this way the body and its embarrassments are rendered safe, abstract, subdivided and scientific.

The body in care is, if anything, more silenced. As we noted in relation to touch, there is no comparable discourse to that of nursing theory with which to describe the processes of care. These practices remain in a zone of silence. As a result careworkers receive little help in dealing with them from their managers or their organisations. Diamond in his vivid ethnographic account of becoming a nursing home aide recounts the difficulty such evasions can pose for new workers. In California, aides are required to receive training, but their male trainer was an ex-nurse and, keen to professionalise the area, emphasised medical knowledge (the student aides were forced to struggle with anatomy) and technical language ('Don't say touching, say tactile communication') (Diamond 1992: 26). Soiled linen was to be 'thrown away', in other words sent to the laundry, but before this could be done the crap and vomit had to be scraped off, a process obscured by his dismissing, distancing language. Despite such 'training', Diamond found himself wholly at a loss when he arrived at the nursing home to be faced with a patient mired in his own shit. Careworkers are on their own in these areas, they either learn by catching sight of others or developing techniques of their own. Either way, their practice is rendered invisible, something beyond the limits of official discourse.

To some degree careworkers concur in this implicit valuation of their work. In describing it they tend to play down the aspect of bodywork, and emphasise 'care' instead. Though it is the body element that marks personal care off from mere domestic cleaning (something that careworkers feel they have moved above in terms of status), it is not the element that they stress. Rather they emphasise the emotional and interpersonal aspects, and the skills required to negotiate and maintain these. These are the most enjoyable and personally rewarding elements; and the parts they want to fore-ground.

As part of this, careworkers were sometimes circumspect when exposing the realities of their work to public view, as the following exchange illustrates:

INTERVIEWER: How do you find dealing with that [faeces], is it difficult?

JAY: *Interesting* (laughter) – it depends where they put it!

Her use of 'interesting' was partly irony but also contained a sense of guarded constraint in exposing these aspects of the work. As a colleague added:

PAT: They all guess, they all know the sort of job you do, don't they—

JAY: That's right.

PAT: I mean you don't go into details, but they just – I mean different people say: 'Oh, I couldn't do that.'

Bates and Lee-Treweek report a similar reticence among careworkers in exposing the realities of their work to the wider world (Bates 1993, Lee-Treweek 1998).

Dealing with dirt and disgust

Modern society as we noted in Chapter 2 rests on a conception of the individual as discrete, contained and separate, and for these reasons incontinence and other forms of unboundedness pose particular difficulties for modern sensibility (Öberg 1996, Lawton 1998). Carework is about dealing with human waste: shit, pee, vomit, sputum; and as such involves managing dirt and disgust. Miller (1997) in his analysis of disgust argues that it is the most visceral of emotions. The idiom of disgust evokes the sensory experience. Taste is the core sensation, mouth the core location and rejection via spitting and vomiting the core actions – actions repeated in our facial expression of disgust. Disgust is rooted in fear of contamination, whether directly through oral incorporation or touching, or more remotely through visual images or moral pollution. Societies vary in what they regard as disgusting or taboo, and in their overall threshold of disgust. Miller argues, echoing Douglas, that the more rule-dense a culture is around food, class, bodily comportment, the lower this threshold is likely to be. For Douglas dirt is matter out of place (Douglas 1966, 1970). It is a by-product of order and classification: where there is dirt there is system. Miller accepts this account, but argues that it is insufficient to capture the element of squeamishness in our responses; and it does not allow for certain recurrences cross-culturally in what is deemed disgusting. Disgust, Miller argues, is rooted in the organic, and above all in the bodily. Disgusting things are slimey, oozing, slithering, moist, clinging; not dry, cold or hard. Disgust is also closely related to other people. Our capacity for self pollution is limited, and it is other people's dirt that concerns us most strongly. Miller believes that disgust rules mark the boundary of the self. Relaxing them characterises privacy, intimacy and caring. Disgust, he argues, plays a complex and possibly necessary relationship in sex and love, and part of the pleasure and peril of sex lies, he believes, in transgressing the prohibitions around the body, and this includes suspension of the rules of disgust.

If we explore the aspects the workers found hardest to cope with, they clearly reflect the category systems described above. Dealing with incontinence was recurringly identified as the most difficult thing to manage. Smell was also hard to bear, and for reasons that echo Lawton's analysis; it had an all-pervasive, stomach-turning quality that lingered about the person:

SUSAN: Someone in a mucky bed, you know, you just – you can put all the protective clothing on, gloves, your plastic apron and everything, but you sometimes feel unclean.

VICKY: The smell stays with you.

Beyond that, individuals varied in what they found difficult. Sharon could not cope with teeth: 'Give me a dirty bum any day than teeth.' Others respondents chimed in:

PETRA: Toenails is mine. I don't like them.

(All speak at once)

VAL: Washing feet and legs when the skin is flaking off, that always gets to me.

TRACEY: What gets to me is when they're coughing up phlegm and put it in a bowl.

(Groans all round.)

Other interviews expanded on the list: 'one thing I can't do is if they need their noses blowing'; 'false teeth'; 'when you hear somebody being sick, you never get used to it, I don't think, anyway'. All share a common source of disgust in the category system recounted by Miller and Douglas. It is other people's bodies and especially the by-products of bodies, or the parts of bodies that are anomalously connected, that are the main focus of revulsion.

Carework as 'dirty work'

So far we have treated carework as dirty work in the obvious way. But carework is so in a second, more sociological sense, also. The term was developed by Hughes and others to cover degrading tasks that are integral to society, but that society does not want to acknowledge, and are by common consent hidden. Emerson and Pollner (1976) extended the term to cover breaches of the moral order at work, encompassing aspects of the job that are shameful, disliked and counter to the self image of the worker. Psychiatric work they argue abounds with dirty work because its day-to-day realities are in conflict with the therapeutic ideal, and they cite getting rid of drunks and derelicts from the psychiatric clinic as part of the dirty work of mental health nursing, something that has to be done, but no one wants to be seen doing.

Dirty work is managed by society through a variety of strategies: by delegating distasteful tasks to lower level staff; by hiding the activity from view; and by otherwise bracketing off the work mentally and socially. Carework illustrates all these. As we noted, the basic bed and bodywork of nursing is commonly delegated to the most junior staff, and dirty work transferred down the occupational hierarchy from nurses to careworkers. Dirty work is also hidden from view. Much bodywork takes place behind the screens and in the back bedrooms of institutions. We owe to Lawler and her path-breaking analysis in *Behind the Screens* (1991), the important perception that this work is obscured not only to protect the privacy of the patient, but also the status and public esteem of the worker. Bodywork is potentially demeaning work, and nurses go off stage to perform it. It may involve inflicting embarrassing or painful procedures; and this needs to be hidden if the image of the nurse is to be maintained. In a similar way Lee-Treweek's account of carework-ers in a residential home, shows how aspects of the work that are at odds with the caring image are managed spatially by being confined to the privacy of the bedrooms (Lee-Treweek 1994). It is here that the basic work of washing, ordering and at times disciplining residents takes place. This 'dirty work' of care is hidden in order that the institution can display the 'product' of its caring regime in the form of the 'lounge standard' patient. Carework in people's own homes requires less in the way of such spatial stratagems since it is by its nature more hidden.

Fundamentally, carework is 'dirty work' because it deals with aspects of life that society, especially modern secular society with its ethic of material success and its emphasis on youth and glamour, does not want to think about: decay, dirt, death, decline, failure. Careworkers manage these aspects of life on behalf of the wider society, ensuring they remain hidden, tidied away into the obscurity of institutions or private homes.

Negotiating the aging body

As we have noted earlier, modern western culture provides us with few images of aging bodies. As a result for some careworkers, particularly the younger ones, the sight of old bodies was a novel and to some degree shocking experience. Sophie found seeing old people naked: 'weird and I just had to stop myself staring at people, because I hadn't really seen ... because you don't really see people naked'. She was surprised at the variety of aging:

> They're so different. Some of them I think they're not ... so different. They're old and they look different from me but I don't know why, what is different, cos they weren't that saggy or that wrinkled or whatever. Whereas some of them if they've got arthritis they get very twisted and some of them really are very wrinkled.... I think people age really differently.

Zara also found naked old bodies a bit of a shock, particularly:

> Like you know, vaginal area and they don't have any hair or it falls off and then you're seeing the whole thing for what it is, you know. That's the only thing that really surprised me really. That's it, cos I just didn't think that hair would, you know, fall off there, and the breasts saggy, you know, and really sag and stuff.

It was noticeable how as a young woman her comments focused on sexual areas. In contemplating old bodies, she implicitly reflected on her own body and on issues of sexual attractiveness and its demise. 'It was a shock how, you know, I look at a person's body and say gosh their body was like mine and look what it deteriorates to.'

Caring for aging bodies means confronting one's own aging. Sophie explained how: 'at first it made me scared of getting old because I thought I don't want to get these things wrong with me or be stuck in my house on my own.' Though the younger workers laughed and joked in the interview about slathering cream on their bodies to keep old age and its wrinkles away, the issue was for most of them a remote one. Aging remained a mystery, something that was hard to grasp and that did not by and large directly impact on their lives. For them the distance between the aging bodies of their clients and their own bodies was too great to be able to make sense of. Barry who was twenty-eight explained: 'It is so distant. It's something which happens to other people but not to myself yet. I know it's bad, or stupid, or short-sighted, but it's the way I feel.'

Many experienced old people as a fixed category – as if they had always been old – and though they knew intellectually that they had once been young, they found it hard to grasp this on an emotional level. The one thing that did bring them up short were the photographs. Barry described one client who had been a professional footballer and who showed him his photographs: 'A big shock there, because I've always known him to be that way there, you know, he was sort of in his mid eighties, and I was imagining him being that way ever since the year dot.'

For Joshua reflecting on photographs raised the issue of his own future:

> They'll show you their married pictures in their younger days, how they used to be, you know you think, oh this man was a soldier, he was an RAF officer or so energetic. And now here he is and I have to bath him, he has no more strength. Am I going to be like this too when I get old, you know? You think of all those things ... it worries me .

The older careworkers identified more directly with the aging process and its impact on their own bodies. But it offered a glimpse into a personal future that was discouraging and unwelcome; and though they accepted it, many chose to push such thoughts away.

How do careworkers cope with bodywork?

Mostly careworkers accept that dealing with human waste is part of the job, and that they have to buckle to and suppress any sense of disgust:

> When Mrs Jones isn't quite so well one day, and you've got diarrhoea from the toilet to the front door, you know. You've got to be able to have a bit of a stomach for the job to actually be able to clear that up.

Some workers internalised the situation and managed their feelings by thinking themselves into the position of a recipient of care. Others consciously reordered the client as a baby – sweet, innocent of intent in making a mess, and vulnerable. Though such techniques could help the worker, they underlie the general infantilisation of older people. Some workers saw dealing with dirt as part of women's inevitable role in life, linking it back to motherhood: 'true there is some dirty aspect of it, but as a woman, you know, you don't bother.'

Stella, the New Age-influenced worker, struggled with the essential ambiguities of bodywork in her sense of revulsion mixed with a wish never to reject the client as a person:

> I think ... there's a part of me that just if something is difficult to look at, difficult to touch I almost feel like I want to embrace it just so that, just because I rejected it so fully you know. It's just the person ... I don't want to feel that revulsion for another human being.

Avoiding direct language is one of the techniques deployed by careworkers in negotiating the body taboos. Careworkers described how they chatted away on the surface while getting over the more difficult or embarrassing aspects in silence. In this way naming the unnameable could be avoided; and language was used to distract and ease rather than to express. Jokes were also a useful distraction.

SUSIE: If you have a joke with them.
MOIRA: You get things done.
SUSIE   You're getting it done before they realise because they're busy laughing.

Humour was a means of coping, both for themselves and the client:

> We joke – I joke, specially if you're actually washing them and they start having a motion and, you know, you say: 'Oh, we've got a surprise here – one minute!' You know, but you just, you can't do it any other way really.

The body and humour are closely linked: dirty jokes, sexual innuendo, 'lavatory' humour – the body is the focus of all these. Mulkay sees discordance and incongruity as at the heart of humour; jokes occur where the single vision of the serious, official account is disrupted by the intrusion of other parallel interpretations and realities (Mulkay 1988). Douglas similarly sees jokes as generated by ambiguity in the social system (Douglas 1975). The body is a ripe source of this, partly because in Douglas's system, it is the symbolic embodiment of the social order generally, and partly because there is an inevitable discordance between the aspirations of formal social life and the desires and failings of the body. The more formal the occasion, the more embarrassing or humorous the body's lapse. In the case of carework, joking was largely used as a means of easing situations that were otherwise embarrassing.

Sometimes, however, the joking was less kindly. In one or two of the group interviews where respondents were more at ease and less concerned to present an idealised account, a different, harsher tone emerged, one of sardonic humour in which 'horror stories' were shared as part of a collective release of feeling in which the solidarity of the workgroup was asserted. Mostly these related to sexual incidents, but the disgusting habits of clients were also recounted. Desiree joked how some of her clients were obsessed with their bowel function, demanding that workers give them suppositories: 'one morning he had two and it wasn't working and he wanted me to put my hands up there and help it along. I told him no way, I'm not doing that.' The group, continuing the vein recounted other cases:

DESIREE: And Mr Jones he takes medicine every single night, to go, so in the morning you sit him on the commode and he has to, you have to be there 'til he's done something.

TONI: Yeah and he must have a look at it.

DESIREE: Yeah, you have to show it to him. Honestly! If you throw it away without him knowing, there's a big argument. He'll say, half, quarter or a full load. Every morning, that's what I'm faced with at nine o'clock in the morning, every single morning.

Workers do not necessarily lose their sense of disgust or their underlying feelings of resentment and anger at what they are required to do. These were predominantly black workers caring for upper middle class white people, and the interview was shot through with tensions in relation to 'race' and class that were reworked into bodily expression. In these more transgressive interviews elements of disgust were not hidden but used against clients.

Bounded intimacy

Carework has a curiously intimate character. Direct physical contact, access to nakedness and the sharing of bodily processes are all powerful mediators of intimacy, containing a capacity to create closeness and dissolve boundaries between people. It is, however, a form of intimacy that is not necessarily sought or enjoyed by those involved. This is most obvious from the perspective of the cared-for person who in accepting body care is required to enter into a relationship of physical and personal exposure that is often unwelcome. But it applies also to the careworkers also who can find the emotional and physical closeness of carework something that they want to resist. The process is most visible in relation to the emotional aspects of carework, and we will explore this more fully in the next chapter. But it has a bodily dimension also. Careworkers can find the physical intimacy of care too strong, and they sometimes take steps to maintain bodily distance. Roz reflected on how she found washing a person in the bath, where there was a barrier provided by the side of the bath and the water, easier than the more intimate process of getting them dry, where contact was more direct and involved the whole body:

> I think that part of the bathing is more embarrassing than actu-
> ally being in the water ... if you're drying somebody you're
> drying them all over ... if somebody's sitting in a bath you're
> usually standing or kneeling by the side of them, when they're
> out of the bath they're actually usually standing up and I don't
> only think it's touch cos touch can be in the bath, I think it's that,
> it's more likely a physical contact and nothing between you,
> you've got the side of the bath, you've got the water in the bath,
> you haven't when they're out of the water and they're holding
> onto the sink or whatever, it's you and that person.

The desire to put limits on the physical intimacy of the work arose most strongly in relation to the negativities of the body. Careworkers have little or no symbolic protection against the polluting nature of their work, unlike nurses who are traditionally invested with a special purity in managing the body and who are able to draw on their quasi-religious status symbolised in the habit-like uniform (Littlewood 1991, Wolf 1988, Bashford 2000). Careworkers by contrast do not by-and-large wear uniforms and their presentation is homely rather than distant or professional (something that was liked by clients). One way in which they do protect themselves is through the use of gloves.

Gloves

Nearly all the careworkers in the study used gloves when bathing clients, and most of the agencies required this. At the simplest level gloves protected workers from some of the less attractive aspects of the job: 'it's nice not to get somebody's faeces under your fingernails'. However, the gloves clearly had other, more symbolic meanings, that went beyond the rationale of hygiene. They provide an example of the processes explored by Douglas in relation to food avoidance whereby 'modern' scientific explanations in terms of hygiene are used to explain practices that have their roots in social categories and symbolism (Douglas 1966). Gloves were used by workers to protect themselves from the full intimacy of bathing work and to put up a barrier of professionalism between the client and the worker.

Sophie, a young worker in London reflected the complex of feelings she had about using gloves:

> When they first said we had to wear gloves, I kind of thought, you know, that's a bit weird sort of thing, a bit, I don't know, I didn't, I thought the clients might feel funny that we thought they were dirty, that we didn't want to touch them sort of thing, but when [the manager] explained it to me why we wore them then I thought it was ok and when it came to actually doing the baths and having the gloves I was really glad to have them on.

Part of the intimacy of carework is that it involves direct skin-to-skin contact with older people. Sophie was surprised by the impact of this on her:

> It was really weird when you feel the skin. Sometimes you budge them with your arm and you feel their skin, but actually to feel someone's skin it's quite different than having the gloves over your hand. It's *much* more intimate.

She felt more at ease wearing gloves particularly where the client was a man:

> with men in particular ... I appreciate wearing them ... you know they might get into it having a nice girl rubbing their back with bare hands ... Having the gloves, it's kind of like wearing a badge saying: I am here for a reason, this is what I'm doing. I'm not just here with you naked, washing you ... I felt better about it.

Sophie's feelings were fairly typical. Gloves operated as a mark of professionalism and distance; they underlined the limited character of this kind of touching; and they protected the worker from a contact that was too direct and too intimate.

Gloves however also bear a symbolic charge, evoking a sense that the person being handled is contaminated. Putting on gloves, protective clothing and masks are all part of the repertoire of frightening, symbolic acts. The use of gloves has been particularly emotive in relation to people with AIDS/HIV; and when the New York police drew on the gloves to deal with gay demonstrators, the messages were strong and clear, and 'take off the gloves' became a rallying call for activists. Some of the sense of this symbolism was caught when one careworker recounted an incident when she and a colleague had gone in to an elderly woman who was not expecting them, and who usually had a cup of tea before her bath, but when she saw them come in, drawing on their gloves and aprons, became upset and disturbed. The story conveyed some of the visceral response that putting the gloves on can evoke: nightmare images of being taken away, or of being dealt with in a frightening alienating way. Careworkers are aware of this, and sometimes feel guilty as a result.

Bodily intimacy: eating, excreting

The desire of careworkers to put boundaries on the intimacy of the work could be detected also in their deployment of exclusionary practices in relation to eating and excreting. We are little accustomed in western society to ideas of eating together as socially or ritually threatening. The dominant discourse is one of conviviality in which eating is experienced in terms of enjoyment and sharing, and commensality – the binding together of people in eating – viewed positively. Other cultures, however, interpret such practices differently; and eating with those of a lower caste, or a different social grouping, can threaten ritual or social impurity. Douglas (1966) argues that all bodily orifices represent danger in the social system, points where the boundaries of social categorisation are under threat. Eating involves a literal incorporation of food, and with that an incorporation of the social connection also. These themes though present are muted in the west. In relation to excretion, the official western account is once again a silent one. Below it, however, exists a series of unofficial practices that suggest that these themes retain a resonance. Institutions like day centres or hospitals where staff refuse to eat with residents or establish their own staff toilet, organisations where promotion is rewarded with a key to the executive washroom, separate facilities in general, all point to an undercurrent of such processes. Sharing the bodily functions implies a form of equality.

Careworkers display aspects of this in relation to their clients. Some, for example, made a point of not eating in the homes of clients.

Though this was expressed in terms of hygiene (not irrelevant in the context of how some older people chose to or were forced to live) what underlay the feeling were social and emotional connections. Eating in the house of a favoured or special client was not rejected.

DESIREE: I've never done that, [eaten in client's house] me I've never done that.
(General chorus of no)
DESIREE: Just want to do my job and get out of their place.

But for a client who was a special favourite even the dirtiness of their house did not matter, as Evie explained:

EVIE: I had this client and his flat was just, pest control should have been called in. Filthy, cobwebs, fungus, everything, well once I got the cups and that, I used to sit on the bed and have a cup of tea and I got very close to that man, very close do you know what I mean like quite happy drinking his tea, eating out of his fridge if it was in a package you know what I mean and he offer it to me.
INTERVIEWER: But that's because you were quite close to him?
EVIE: Yeah, *if I don't like the person I wouldn't stay.*

So shared ingestion is about closeness and not just hygiene.

Diamond's account of the views of a fellow nursing home aide also illustrate this relational quality:

She told me in all seriousness that 'some shit don't stink'. I asked her to explain a bit more what she meant. As she was teaching me how to make a bed, she made it perfectly clear: 'It depends on if you like 'em and they like you, and if you know them pretty well; it's hard to clean somebody new, or somebody you don't like. If you like them, it's like your baby.' A bit later she made reference to a man with whom she had had to struggle every day: 'But now take Floyd, that bastard, that man's shit is foul.' Through her explanation it became clear that the work is not a set of menial tasks, but a set of social relations in which the tasks are embedded

(Diamond 1988: 49)

Diamond is arguing that even the most directly physical aspect of the task – whether the shit smells – is mediated by the nature of the relationship.

Some careworkers would not go to the lavatory in a client's home, even where they had cleaned it themselves:

TONI: You can't even go to the toilet

DESIREE: That's it, you can't go toilet, that's the big problem. I find that I hold myself 'til I get home in the evening, which is not good, but that's what I do.

INTERVIEWER: Why is that?

DESIREE: 'Cos some of the toilets are – you might be cleaning them but I just can't bring myself to go to them or – or you feel you don't wanna use people's toilets. No.

DAWN: There's probably about three people's—

DESIREE: If I go to Mrs Mansfield's I must admit, yeah, I use her toilet, 'cos it's nice and cosy and clean, but I couldn't use Mr Jones' toilet. Well some people they get offended if you ask if you can use the toilets, like they don't want you to use them.

DAWN: I think it's embarrassing when you have to ask a man if you can use the toilet, you know, I feel embarrassed if I'm in a man's house and I want to go.

DESIREE: It's difficult 'cos being a woman you know you have the time of the month and you have to use the toilet, it's, it's just difficult if you're in a man's house and you have to go in your bag [laughter]. Terrible.

The unease had a sexual element in it, rooted in embarrassment about periods. But it also suggested the desire to maintain distance. Sharing a lavatory seemed to imply a closeness or equality that was not wanted, a reminder that they – the careworkers – also had bodily needs like those that the clients were forced to expose.

Sex and the careworker

Personal care occurs on the borderland of sexuality, and dealing with unwanted sexual behaviour is one of the minor tasks of carework. Sometimes male clients tried it on:

> He was always trying to get us to wash his private parts ... and I think I did it the first time cos I was quite new, and Hazel said to me, you never have to do that really ... He could do it, and I realised this when he turned the shower on. I thought, if he can do that, then he can do it. He's just trying it on.

Men who persist are typically transferred to a male careworker.

As with sexual harassment more widely, the character of the exchange is defined in the fine texture. Comments that from one person are just part of the give and take of jokes, a flirty spin on the exchange, can cause unease or a sense of threat from another. By and large the careworkers took sexual incidents in their stride:

'it's just a bit of fun.'

'We can handle them, can't we?'

'We need longer skirts (laughter)'

'cheeky ... they just like to egg you on.'

Sophie, an attractive flirty young woman, accustomed to being the centre of male eyes, watched what she wore: 'I've got a skirt on today and I did check my rota to make sure I didn't have any saucy men that I'm visiting'. So potential difficulties were got round through the language of sauciness. Another woman made a joke of it:

One man I used to go to used to reach out for me and try to grab me ... and I just used to make some kind of joke of it, you know. I used to say something like: 'Well you should really have my sister here, 'cos I've got two fried eggs' .... And he just used to grin at me, no teeth in and – and the next day he'd be OK.

Sometimes the incidents were more embarrassing or unpleasant, and workers were made to feel uneasy and insecure. Clients would brush up against them or make nasty personal remarks. Recounting 'horror tales' to fellow workers was one way of dealing with this:

DAWN: I had one man once and he was standing there and his willy was sticking out and he said 'Oh, I need attention, I need attention' (laughter) and he was holding two sticks (laughter)—
DESIREE: Oh my God! Attention! The things we have to put up with.
DAWN: I said 'Well I can't give you attention' I said, 'I've got too much to do here, so—
DESIREE: Just say 'Stick it in the bottle.'

It is important to note the tone of this exchange and the sense of resentment among the workers at what they have to put up with.

Recounting such tales gives workers a chance to assert themselves against clients, to turn the situation round and use it against perpetrators. In a similar way workers sometimes used impotence to denigrate clients who attempted sexual contact. As Desiree said: 'They all stay still, nothing moves, so I know they're quite dead (general laughter)'. Ultimately the women knew they could control the situation because clients were weak and did not offer a serious sexual threat. As Hazel remarked: 'They're only old. It doesn't matter.'

Bodywork as gendered work

Resonating through the concept of bodywork is the issue of gender. There are a complex set of reinforcing influences that together construct bodywork as female. First, these are tasks that are naturalised in the bodies and persons of women. Women have traditionally represented the Body in culture (Jordanova 1989, Lupton 1994). They have been presented as more bodily than men, bound up in and defined by the processes of reproduction, and prey to the shifting tides of emotion. Women also represent the Body in terms of male desire, the form of desire hegemonic in culture. They thus come to represent sexuality itself, something that can be controlled through the control of women's bodies. Confining desire (at least in its legitimate forms) and the needs of the body to the domestic sphere allows the public world to be constructed as disembodied, rational and male. A simple example of the consequences of this can be seen in the problems faced by women MPs in breastfeeding in the House of Commons.

Bodywork is also intimately linked with women's bodily lives through motherhood and nurturance. Because women do this work for babies and children, these activities are generalised as female. Ungerson (1983) has suggested that the association of women with bodywork and in particular with dealing with body wastes reflects a wider sense of women as polluted. Women, she argues, are assigned by culture to deal with these matters because they themselves belong to the realm of the body, its fluxes and wastes. We saw how one careworker saw dealing with waste as something that was an ordinary part of women's work.

Presenting carework as natural for women also reinforces the perception of it as unskilled. As such, it does not require training or qualifications, nor justify the better wages that skilled work traditionally enjoys. Though bodywork is poorly regarded in terms of pay and employment esteem, it also often extravagantly praised, particularly by men who do not have to do it. Home helps, like nurses, are traditionally described in glowing terms, and this often includes a sense that the speaker could not – that is, would not want to – do this work. There are similarities in the way in which mothers and housewives are presented in conservative discourse: their work is sidelined, lowly regarded and unsupported, and yet at the same time presented as of supreme value. Porter interprets this in terms of the patriarchal feminine which, while seeming to value and praise female work, in fact reinforces female subordination (Porter 1992).

Lastly women's association with bodywork derives from the greater freedom that women are accorded in their access to bodies compared with men. Hegemonic masculinity constructs men as sexually predatory; and limits are placed on male access to bodies, male or female (Connell 1995). Female sexuality by contrast is presented as passive, waiting arousal and more limited in its scope. This, together with the dominance of the maternal model, means that women are allowed greater leeway in performing the transgressive acts of bodycare without their being constructed as threatening or sexual, as might be the case with a male worker. We saw in Chapter 6 how the work of male careworkers is circumscribed, and how in general males do not give personal care to women, at least in their own homes. Women careworkers by contrast are sanctioned to do this work on the bodies of both men and women, and this reinforces the concept of carework as gendered work. We will return to this further in the next chapter.

Conclusion

In this chapter we have explored the nature of carework through the medium of a concept of bodywork. This brings a number of benefits. First it enabled us to foreground aspects of the work that have previously been downplayed. Carework is fundamentally about bodywork, and manipulating, cleaning and caring for bodies is at the heart of the activity, though our traditions of analysis have some-times obscured this fact. Seeing carework as bodywork also enables us to reassert the mundane and concrete character of the activity, its hands-on, down-to-earth nature, compared with some of the more aetherialising accounts of 'care'.

Bodywork is work that takes place behind the screens of social life, and it is often hidden, silenced work, occurring below the level of the official account. Workers receive little guidance in this area. What official discourse does exist is often unhelpful and at odds with the day-to-day realities of the work. Deploying the concept of bodywork by contrast enables us to bring some definition to the field, and to link it to other parallel areas of work. We noted how careworkers choose not to emphasise these aspects of their work in public, and this is despite the fact that it is the bodywork element that marks personal care off from the low-level domestic cleaning that they feel they have moved above. The aspects that they prefer to foreground are the 'care' ones, the emotional and interpersonal side of the work. In doing this they follow a wider dematerialising tendency within the ranking of work whereby status is measured by distance from the bodily. High status actors protect and maintain their positions by distancing techniques, by time limited contact and by the use of divisions of labour, particularly those reinforced by gender, to bracket off the activity socially. At a simple level, bodywork takes place behind the screens to protect the privacy of clients. But as we saw in relation to Lawler's account of nursing, this is not the whole story, and bodywork is also hidden to protect the status of the worker.

Carework is ambivalent work, dealing with the taboo and diffi-cult area of the human body and its wastes. It manages the negativities of the body and the aspects of human physicality that modern society has become increasingly intolerant of in the pursuit of postmodern dreams of autonomy, boundedness and youthful success. Carework is poorly regarded and demeaned work, performed by workers who have little purchase on the labour market. It comes low in career choices. And yet at the same time, it is often praised and lauded by the wider society which links it to the special status of motherhood and to the saintly virtues of love and care. What makes the workers special and saintly is that they do – or rather 'give' – this intimate and close care, and yet this is also what makes the work demeaning and of low esteem. These tensions are resolved – or rather contained – within the person of the woman worker. Her body both expresses and contains these ambivalences. In the case of nursing this is managed by means of the symbolism of nursing culture. Careworkers however have none of this protective status, and they have few symbolic means of protecting themselves against the nature of the work.

But bodywork also encompasses the body-pleasing and body-enhancing trades that are about creating zones of wellbeing and pleasure, in which touch and shared intimacy can be part of the treatment. The bodywork of care can contain something of this. We saw in Chapter 3 how bathing for older and disabled people could involve aspects of pleasure and sensuousness – the feeling of water being poured over the person, the luxury of shower foam, the warmth and lightness of the water – and one worker at least saw the links between her work and New Age-style therapeutics. There are, however, limits to this. Careworkers do get close to their clients as part of the work, but this closeness contains its own tensions. As we saw in relation to massage, bodywork occupies an ambiguous position, and pleasure and touch have an uncertain status as part of work. Recipients of care concurred in this, finding it difficult to acknowledge pleasure in touch. Workers were themselves ambivalent about these aspects of the work, preferring to emphasise the social and emotional aspects of closeness rather than the bodily ones.

Lastly, bodywork creates tensions around intimacy and closeness and we saw how careworkers sometimes put limits on the bodily intimacy of the work, putting up barriers like gloves against its direct physicality and avoiding activities like eating that underwrote shared bodily existence. Keeping a distance was also a means of underlining the asymmetrical character of the relationship, in which the worker was clearly in charge. Bodywork creates an ambivalent form of closeness in which the power dynamics can tip over either way. We saw this in relation to prostitution and the demeaned status of the body servant, in which to be subordinated in such an intense, direct and bodily way carried a particularly high charge. But the reverse is also true. Bodywork is a prime site for the exercise of bio-power. To establish control over the bodies of people is to make them subordinate in a particularly demeaning way, and there is a strongly coercive element running through the symbolism of bodycare, in potential at least. We will return to these themes in Chapter 9.

8 Carework as emotional labour

In the last chapter we analysed carework as a species of bodywork, drawing out some of its recurring features as gendered labour. In this chapter we turn to the other half of the equation, exploring the less tangible aspects of care – those encompassing feelings and emotion – exploring carework as a form of emotional labour. Carework is more often interpreted in terms of the debate on care. This arose initially out of the analysis of informal care, though it has its roots also in debates within moral and political philosophy concerning the differential responses of men and women to moral obligation (Gilligan 1982, Finch and Groves 1983, Ungerson 1987, 1990, Lewis and Meredith 1988, Larabee 1993, Parker 1993, Tronto 1993, Twigg and Atkin 1994). Though originally concerned with the private sphere, work on care has increasingly crossed over to encompass care as paid work (Graham 1991, Ungerson 1993). The classic example of this is nursing, and in the last part of the chapter we will explore the ways in which the element of care within nursing has been interpreted as part of a wider analysis of gender.

Emotional labour

Emotional labour as a concept was developed by Hochschild, and has been extended by James and others (Hochschild 1983, James 1989, 1992). For Hochschild, emotional labour involves both working on and through the feelings of others, with the aim of producing an effect on their emotional state. It is a central feature of most service work, and arises where there is direct face-to-face contact between the worker and the client/customer. Hochschild developed the concept in relation to female flight attendants whose work revolves around attending to the personal needs and feelings of male passengers. Emotional labour involves close attention to another, interpreting and responding to their needs; and to work properly, it requires staff to go beyond a mere formulaic response and give something of themselves. Emotional labour demands that workers control their own feelings, and it may extend to displaying emotions that are at odds with their inner state. James has extended the concept in relation to work within the hospice and in doing so has identified a number of its features. Emotional labour is often an invisible, unrecorded element of work – something that is assumed but not openly acknowledged. It can be hard, emotionally draining work, and yet usually regarded as unskilled, something that workers, particularly women workers, 'just do'. It is gendered work 'that capitalises on the qualities and capabilities a women has gained by virtue of having lived her life as a woman' (Davis and Rosser, quoted in James 1989: 31). James believes that it is, in fact, something that can be learnt, and that its exercise is open to all who have an interest in, or obligation to, acquire these skills.

Seeing carework as emotional labour brings certain advantages. First it avoids some of the conceptual ambiguity that attaches to the word 'care'. Care as a concept grew out of the analysis of informal care, and it aimed to describe the complex of activities, feelings and obligations that are involved in the support of individuals, usually family members. Emotional labour by contrast allows one to separate out the feeling element from other strands, and in particular from the norms and values that attach to kinship and family obligation. Emotional labour also avoids some of the difficulties around the halo effect that attaches to the word 'care'. Care in English is a notoriously slippery term that elides normative and descriptive elements. It is almost impossible to separate care from aspects of love, and with it from warmth and value. It is difficult to resist the ethic of love (with its long undertow from the influence of Christianity in western culture), and this is one of the reasons why we have difficulty in conceptualising love adequately in sociology. Emotional labour by contrast has the advantage of greater analytic detachment. This makes it easier to see it as part of the labour process. James (1992) argues that hospice work is better seen as a category of work-place based health care than as an extension of family responsibility, and that tensions arise when attempts are made to apply the model of family care to the work place. She believes that there is a basic discordance. Lee-Treweek (1998) similarly argues that the feminist account of care deriving from informal care within the family distorts our understanding of paid carework, failing to engage with the ways in which it is a work activity shaped by similar forces to those affecting other service occupations.

Emotional labour needs to be set in the context of the wider intellectual enterprise concerning the analysis of emotion within society, particularly as an element in work. Accounts of organisations, particularly those rooted in the Weberian tradition, have until recently ignored the role of emotions at work, either writing them out altogether or perceiving them as disruptive and improper intrusions into the work setting. (There are parallels here with the treatment of the body within the rationalistic tradition discussed in Chapter 1.) Emotion is regarded as sitting uneasily with the bureaucratic values of impartiality, efficiency, predictability. By contrast, Fineman argues that emotions are central to organisations because they are fundamental to all social order, constitutive of the day-to-day realities that we take for granted in our working and organisational lives. Emotional labour is a general feature of much work, and it is a mistake to associate it solely with routinised service work. More esteemed – and male – work-like management also contains a significant element of emotional labour (Finemen 1993, Hochschild 1993).

Hochschild presents emotional labour as something that is potentially damaging to the worker. Because the feelings involved are at the command of the organisation, the work estranges the worker from herself, undermining authenticity, so that the mask begins to eat into the face. Adkins (1995) in her account of sexualised work (the study centred on barmaids and staff in the leisure industry) emphasised how a particular sort of femininity was enjoined on workers by the organisation, and she identifies the oppressive character of such roles. There is a recurring problem, however, in the analysis of service work that aspects that academics identify as exploitative are often enjoyed and valued by the workers; and one of the attractions of service work for many people is precisely the human interaction. For some women banter and flirtation makes the dull work of selling drinks tolerable. Wharton (1993), for example, found that performing emotional labour was related positively to job satisfaction among nurses and bank employees, and was viewed by both as one of the attractions of the work. Accounts of supermarket work make similar points: checkout workers enjoyed the human contact with customers; it lightened and cheered what was otherwise a boring and mechanical task. Many of the same dynamics apply to home care. What the workers valued most were the human interactions they had with clients. Emotional labour does contain a capacity for alienation, but this is by no means always present, and emotional labour, as we shall see, can be a source of pleasure and enjoyment.

Lee-Treweek in her account of nursing home work extends the concept of emotional labour (though she uses the term emotion work) to include the emotional manipulation deployed by care assistants as part of getting the work done (Lee-Treweek 1996). Emotion work for her is a dynamic mechanism for creating order in a residential setting, involving elements of both nurturance and control. Using emotional skills enables care assistants to get through their work and create order in the home. Workers develop these skills for themselves. They are not part of the official regime of management, but a set of techniques deployed autonomously by workers. Sometimes these techniques run counter to the official care regime of the home, and can be regarded as subversive of it, representing a form of 'resistance' by the workers. Care assistants used emotional techniques to exert control over the conditions of their labour. Through giving and withholding personal warmth, they were able to set up a system of rewards and punishments by means of which the behaviour of residents can be controlled. Residents who resist such emotional manipulation, particularly the infantalising that was a frequent part of it, are labelled 'difficult' by the workers. Their indifference to the emotional bribery of carework threatened the power of the care assistants and was resented by them. Lee-Treweek interprets these relations in terms of Foucault's concept of 'pastoral care' – a mode of power in which the shepherd knows and cares for the flock, giving individual attention to each, and through such processes of care is able to order and command their lives totally. This 'nurturant power' is particularly significant in relation to women, enabling them to exercise power without overtly seeming to do so, and in situations where to do so is not openly legitimate.

Lee-Treweek's extension of the concept of emotion work to encompass these darker, manipulative elements is an important one, that has a wider significance for the role of women in a range of settings, including the family; and it goes some of the way towards redressing accounts that have presented women as powerless, as well as uniquely virtuous. Lee-Treweek shows how women use emotional skills to get their way. 'Care' is not always kind; nor is it always selfless. Women exert power through their skill in manipulating feelings, and they are socialised to develop and hone such abilities. As Baker Miller (1978) points out, emotional acuity and capacity to interpret the moods of others is a characteristic of servants and women: individuals whose formal power is limited. The powerful by contrast do not need to monitor or consult the feelings of those beneath them.

Though Lee-Treweek retains the distinction made by Hochschild between emotional labour and emotional work (emotional labour being non-autonomous and at the behest of the organisation, and emotion work under the personal control of the worker), in common with most writing in this area I will simply use the term emotional labour, but with the proviso that I do not intend always to imply alienation (though such is a possibility), and I do want to retain the capacity, present in Lee-Treweek, of workers using emotion autonomously as a form of manipulation. I also do not want to lose the sense – which I think at times Lee-Treweek does – that these are emotions that are *experienced* by workers and not just used by them. Emotional labour involves emotion on both sides. One of the central tensions of carework is that it involves the worker emotionally in ways that can be painful and exhausting. Careworkers develop strong feelings for their clients, and these can be a source of difficulty as well as reward.

Bathwork as emotional labour

Bathwork displays all the classic features of emotional labour. It requires a direct personal engagement by the worker on a one-to-one basis. The very intimacy of the contact means that emotions are inevitably in play, indeed to perform the work coldly and without emotion is to fail in a central aspect of it. The emotional state of the client is also an important element in the exchange, and careworkers work on the feelings of their clients just as they work on their bodies. This emotional work is, however, never just one-way, and caring creates ties and bonds of affection that act back on the workers.

The rewards of carework are direct and immediate, and few jobs can offer such strong positive feedback. Care is something that brings its own rewards: seeing the pleasure that your help gives; knowing your work is valuable and important to someone, even though society at large does not value it greatly, at least in terms of money or status. This was something that Barry, who was otherwise concerned about the low status of the work, recognised:

> I get enjoyment, I have to admit, that I get enjoyment out of it and pleasure.... seeing the pleasure on somebody's face when you walk through the door first thing in the morning ... The pleasure

of seeing the client's face and knowing that, when you leave, they're happy.

This is the best part of the work. As Janet reiterated you: 'can get a lot back from a grateful client'. Emotional labour was experienced by the workers as one of the prime advantages of the job.

Many workers in the study went to considerable efforts to encourage and cheer their clients; and the accounts of respondents in the study were full of testimonies to their success in doing so. Remaining constantly upbeat and positive, however, can be a strain. As Sophie explained: 'mentally you just feel really zapped ... all this input and often people are depressed or lonely and you're their only visit. So you've got to have all the energy.' Often the worker is the client's only human contact, and this puts special burdens and responsibilities on them: 'They hardly have any visitors and they really look forward to you coming ... you know how important that is to them. So [despite feeling drained] I suppose I put them first.'

As with nursing or hospice work, the emotional labour of care is not just a matter of responding naturally from the heart (though that is the impression that workers aim to convey), it also involves the deployment of skills. Though carework is rarely trained work as such, it is still skilled. It is just that the skills are those built up through experience of life and personal sensitivity. Exercising such skills can be a challenge: gaining the trust of someone who is withdrawn or nervous; encouraging the embarrassed to feel at ease; supporting the depressed, are all skilled tasks. Even difficult and aggressive clients can be a source of satisfaction, as Janet, the manager of a voluntary sector scheme, explained:

> There's a great achievement to manage a difficult client. It's easy to manage the easy ones.... Some people, it's a challenge, you know, and coping and managing with difficult clients ... People can feel really satisfied with themselves afterwards, for a job well done.

Though the workers regard the work as skilled and demanding, they also see it as something that is natural, or at least natural to people like themselves. Careworkers describe themselves as women who are caring by nature and who at some level 'need' to do this sort of work. Softheartedness was identified as a self characteristic. One woman felt that she could be a careworker because it allowed for such feelings – 'there is a need in me to help other people' – but being a nurse required a tougher attitude since nurses 'have to be cruel to be kind'. The workers are aware that not all of them are like this. There are some 'hard girls' who do it just for the money and give very little, but they are disapproved of and perceived as exceptions. Mostly they are thought to work in residential homes. Judy, the manager of home care in Coastville, was clear that genuine warmth and emotion were central to the work: 'You can't be doing carework just for the money. You can't.' She had had one worker whom she felt was just interested in money, signing up to for all hours with various agencies, and juggling and neglecting clients, and so she stopped using her.

Carework, as Janet explained, is intrinsically about emotion; so that the cold careworker, even if super-efficient, can never be a really good carer and she was clear that the best workers offered not just care but 'love':

> You see you can get a very efficient carer. Who will do all the technical and all the things that they're asked to do, but there isn't the rapport there or the emotional contact. I've had carers like that. They're very efficient and all the rest of it, but to me they lack a certain something ... You can get a carer who may not be the best when it comes to the technical side, but they're absolutely wonderful when it comes to the emotional support. The caring they give, you know, I mean genuine caring, well, love really.

The emotion on offer here was 'real'.

In Hochschild's account, emotional labour is damaging to the workers because it erodes authenticity and, through the deep acting it requires, corrupts the capacity to feel. This was not how the careworkers in the study perceived things. Though caring could be emotionally tiring, particularly for a demanding or depressed client, the danger of the work came not from self-estrangement, but from the reality and strength of the ties that it created. Getting attached to clients was an occupational hazard as well as a source of pleasure. Strong feelings were inevitable, particularly where contact was sustained:

SUSIE: Because I know you're not supposed to get attached to people, but you do, you can't help it, because if you weren't a caring sort of person you couldn't do this job, could you?
MAGGIE: No, that's right.

SUSIE: And you do – I mean I've been going to one of my clients for five years – well how can you spend five years at someone's house and not make a friend of them, you know, not get attached to them?

There is a constant struggle to maintain distance:

GILLIAN: You just sort of try and bear back a bit, you know, but sometimes you just can't, especially ...
MAGGIE: You get ever so attached.
GILLIAN: Yeah.
SUSIE: Well you're there doing everything for them, you're there listening to their little problems, aren't you, you're bound to get, aren't you.

Careworkers felt most deeply for those clients who were most reliant on them. Relations with clients who were one half of a couple, or who lived with children, were never as strong or intimate. These individuals had alternative emotional focuses in their lives; and for them help with bathing or personal care was an instrumental and tangential activity. The cases where the workers felt closest to the clients were those where they depended on them most fully. Often these were frail and isolated individuals; and it was this that created the emotional charge. There was a clear 'Tamagotchi' effect to this emotional bonding. Tamagotchi toys rely on a central human truth: that what creates attachment and love is not attractiveness but need. It is the constant care that Tamagotchis require to keep them 'alive' that turns them into powerful sources of emotional bonding. In a similar way, it is the neediness of clients that creates the strong bonds of caregiving.

Being close inevitably creates a capacity to be hurt. Among the hardest things for workers to bear was the active unhappiness of a client. This was particularly difficult where the client made a direct emotional appeal to the worker – the hand on the sleeve and the quavering voice asking them not to leave – but it applied also to the sense of relief once the worker had managed to get away from the pain and unhappiness, out into the sunshine of the street. Some workers felt guilty about their ability to escape, but most recognised that they had to put such thoughts aside. The most successful workers (and they included some whose caring was highly commended by both clients and managers) were those who could switch off their emotions once they had left.

Death was an obvious source of distress, but also produced a wry sense of humour. Again, careworkers had to learn how to set limits on their involvement.

MAGGIE: You harden yourself, don't you – you have to, don't you?
BEA: I think you have to, yes, otherwise you just—
SUSIE: I think one year I felt like, I felt like a professional funeral goer, one year—
MAGGIE: Yes, that's right.
SUSIE: I did, you know. And I felt the people at the crematorium, they must have thought: 'She's here again'.
MAGGIE: Yeah, I've had about four since Christmas (amusement).

Careworkers have to make themselves emotionally open to clients as part of the work. As a result, however, nastiness on behalf of the client is particularly distressing, as the following incident, which also has a sexual element, shows. The careworker recounted how one man kept saying:

'Scrub my back, scrub my back'. Then when I come to do his private parts he says: 'Oh, watch out', he says, you know, 'I'm tender down there', he said. 'How would you like me to take a pair of pliers to your clitoris?' I was absolutely! – I mean there again, I was so gobsmacked I just let it ride. But when I get home I thought: '*If* I tell my husband, he'd go mad'.

The other workers in the group concurred that aggression and nastiness and feeling that you can do nothing right were the hardest things to cope with. One worker said she had a cry in such circumstances, and the others consoled her saying they were the same. This is the reverse side of their emotional support and responsiveness: if the clients seem to attack, dislike, or not value them, it is hard to bear. Another worker in the group recounted how she went to the same man and :

I couldn't see, because he won't let you draw the curtains or turn the light on, and I couldn't see and I think – I have rubber gloves on and I must have caught, I caught him with my finger, and he moaned and I said: 'Well I'm sorry', I said, 'But it's so dark in here, I can't see'. 'Are you bloody blind?' he said.

But then out of the blue, he said 'thanks' and she felt wonderful. These workers are on a rollercoaster of his feelings as a result of their responsiveness and wish to be loved.

Careworkers, because they get their rewards from emotional dependence, can sometimes manipulate the situation to maximise this; and carework contains a constant capacity to increase the dependence of clients; something that the managers were very aware of: 'Some carers, do like to take over people's lives and they do like to do everything for people ... We have carers who say, "Why did you get out of bed before I came to help you? Why did you dress yourself?" '. Paulette Gibson acknowledged that: 'Careworkers get quite dependent on their clients actually, it's a sort of a two-way process.' Skeggs argues that careworkers draw their sense of self esteem from the dependence of others, and this is used to mitigate the otherwise poor estimation of the work (Skeggs 1997).

Very occasionally careworkers felt that clients tried to take advantage of their good natures, pushing them to do more and more. This angered them and was seen as a serious breach of the implicit care contact in which the client was 'needy' and the worker 'caring'. Being genuinely needy or genuinely grateful were important features of an acceptable client. Some clients, however, perhaps encouraged by the new consumerist language in relation to care, took a more contractual even adversarial approach, trying to get the worker to do more as part of extracting more labour for the price. This was much resented:

> When I first started going to this particular client she expected me to do the hoovering and everything in that half an hour sort of thing, and I said to her, it's not on, I can't do it. And she goes, oh you're too lazy to do it, and things like that. So I actually phoned my manager up and I explained and said I don't want to go in there anymore. She's just sort of taking advantage.

Carework as unbounded work

There are obvious affinities between carework and informal, family-based care. Both spheres are strongly associated with women; and many of the tasks, both practical and emotional, are the same. Of itself, this does not pose difficulties for workers. Carework is a commodified form of care, but the careworkers in general did not perceive this as odd or disjunctive. It was work that needed to be done, and that drew on qualities and expertise that they had. For many it was a natural extension of their work in the family. Problems did arise however from the importation into paid work of an unbounded ethic of responsibility that has its roots in the primary bonds of the family. Informal care rests ultimately on the sense of 'being responsible', of doing whatever is necessary, of being the bottom line (Twigg and Atkin 1994). Informal care does, of course, have its limits and it is not devoid of structures of expectation or boundary setting (Finch 1989, Finch and Mason 1993). There is, however, an anti-structural ethic contained within it, and expressed through the ethic of love; and it is the tension between this un-bounded, unstructured ethic and more formal accounts of action that causes many of the difficulties in the analysis of care. When carework is performed under the conditions of waged labour, this anti-structural, totalising ethic of love meets and clashes with the principles of economic rationality and the highly structured, measured conditions of formal employment.

Careworkers in general subscribe to the ethic of care, but are forced to perform their work in the context of wage labour. Their jobs, and the incentives in relation to them, are structured by economic rationality; indeed as we have seen the sector has increasingly been made subject to these principles. The work thus does have clear limits in the sense that the careworkers are only allocated and paid for specific periods of time and often only for certain tasks. This creates tensions for the workers, caught between the personalised demands of the ethic of care and the reality of hourly paid wage labour.

One of the classic features of this tension is the existence of 'extras': work undertaken by staff outside the official schedule of duties. 'Extras' are a recurring feature of home care, and one found across welfare systems (Warren 1988, Sinclair *et al.* 1990, Aronson and Neysmith 1996). Typically they cover things like: taking the client Christmas shopping, making birthday cakes, running round with a plate of Sunday dinner, buying underwear, taking the cat to the vet, bringing a husband round to clear the gutters, popping back in the evening to tuck the person in; and all of these featured in the interviews. Some extras represent things not provided by the welfare system but that are needed or valued by the client; others represent the shortfall between what the system is willing to allocate and what the worker feels is needed. Either way, extras are unrecompensed labour.

Workers are aware of this tension. Working on an hourly basis in an increasingly hard-nosed employment context, they know that 'extras' mean that: 'you're doing it for nothing, aren't you.' But they are still drawn into the dynamic of need and response that gives rise to them. Learning how to put limits and say 'no' is thus an important part of learning to cope with the job. A number of workers recounted how they had forced themselves to come to some balance, realising that the job could take over their lives. One recounted the common experience of giving out her phone number, only to find she was rung at five in the morning: 'you can't possibly do it really, 'cos you have your own life, don't you?' If you are not careful the work takes over everything:

MAGGIE: I used to take four bags of washing home – oh!
BEA: That's what I said ... you've got to cut yourself off because ... it's so easy, you know, to be able to throw their washing in with yours and, you know, and then you—
MAGGIE: It runs over into your life ... All of a sudden you've got another mum or grandma.

It is important to note how this respondent links the engulfing potential of the work to the model of kinship. Responding fully to its dynamic threatens you with an additional set of relatives. Part of the task of carework is to put a limit on these tendencies, and to push back the encroachment of the ethic of care. Women careworkers sometimes used their husbands as a means of doing this, balancing one sort of gendered demand made on them with another. Three workers recounted how their husbands had put their foot down and stopped them doing clients' washing. Another recounted how her husband went mad about the rubbish: 'I do take rubbish home for somebody and I have to smuggle it in and put it in my dustbin 'cos my husband gets so: "Haven't we got enough rubbish of our own?" '

Managers have always been aware of these activities, and in large degree have turned a blind eye. Indeed many, in praising the home care workforce for their dedication and commitment, cite their involvement in extras. This is not seen primarily as an aspect of the work, so much as a result of a personal feature of the workers – their caring and kindly natures. That character is praised – sometimes to the skies – but not rewarded financially. It is regarded as something that arises naturally from their character as caring women. It is not what they *do* but who they *are*. Extras thus represent work that is extracted on the basis of the traditional gender contract, but not officially recognised or recompensed in the formal one.

Care as work is in large degree unrecognised and unrewarded. Because we lack the conceptual means to capture the element of care in work (and indeed more widely within social action), it is frequently overlooked and ignored. As Neysmith and Aronson (1996) comment, the public discourse of home care provision attends to practical task accomplishments that can be charted and counted. Supervisors lack a workplace vocabulary for personalising work and emotional labour so that 'service work job descriptions are limited to task specification while the relationship components of the work remain invisible and unnamed' (1996: 8).

Carework falls into that diffuse category of activities that Tronto (1993) analyses in terms of making, repairing and maintaining our worlds, and this encompasses bodies, selves and environment. This sense of care as a knitting together and repairing of the world – the feminine metaphors of sewing, quilting, mending, tidying are very strong – expresses important aspects: its constant and continuing character; its nature as process; its modest, secondary character, servicing the needs of others. And it finds echo in Balbo's earlier conceptualisation of women's work in terms of piecing together the social fabric, in such a way as to link up its discordant fragments (Balbo 1987). Carework also contains something of this sense: sorting things out, smoothing problems, negotiating difficulties, operating at different levels, bodily, emotional, practical, interpersonal. And they all contribute to the boundless, undefined nature of the work.

Lastly, carework is like other gendered activities such as housework, childcare and nursing where the task is one of sustaining a state and where as a result there is no clear or stable product of the work. The state it creates is fragile, and the work is never done because it can perpetually be undone. This contributes both to the unbounded character of carework, and to the fluidity of its concept of time. As we saw in Chapter 4, though you may schedule a period of time in which to do the task, its accomplishment is never certain, so the time of carework and the time of clock work are never quite the same. This applies both to the bodywork element in care: the constant entropy of leaking bodies; and the emotional dimension. Careworkers find it hard to leave clients who are distressed and need them at that moment. Putting limits on the work whether in terms of time or emotion is often hard; and there is an essentially unbounded character to care.

The emotional labour of carework

There are a series of linked features that characterise the emotional labour of carework, and that have their roots in assumptions about gender. First, this is labour that is only partly visible. Though accepted as central to the job, it is not fully articulated as such. Managerial descriptions of the work, particularly those rooted in the task-specific definitions, frequently gloss over or omit it. Emotion is not part of the rationalistic, bureaucratic account. As a result, this aspect of the work is not fully recompensed. Staff are officially rostered only to do certain things, though they are assumed to do others in addition, unofficially, on their basis of them as caring women. The emotional labour of carework is thus delivered by means of the traditional gender contract, and not reflected or recompensed in the formal one. The ability to do emotional labour is deemed to reside in the character of the workers rather than their training or skills. It is an intangible quality that comes from who they are: good women (with the possibility that they might be bad ones – 'hard girls' – and a hope that these will not have been recruited).

Second, there is an unbounded, limitless character to carework. This derives in part from its unstable nature; the product is constantly in process of being made and unmade. This creates a disjunction between the clock-time of schedules and the process time of need. Caring is also infused with an ethic of love that has an unbounded, anti-structural quality to it. This comes not just from the translation over from the private family sphere of senses of obligation or definitions of caring that emphasise the ultimate responsibility of the carer, but also from the emotional charge of the work that creates bonds that are difficult to resist. Close contact on a one-to-one basis (and we noted in Chapter 6 how this contrasts with residential care) with individuals who are emotionally and physically dependent on the worker can create powerful feelings. Careworkers experience emotions as well as work on them. As a result, putting limits on the demands of the work is a central need, if one is to survive and not be engulfed. Running through all these features is the thread of gender, and in the next section we will explore the ways in which the element of care has been analysed within another occupation that is also constructed around assumptions about gender: nursing.

Caring as gendered work: the example of nursing

Nursing has also wrestled conceptually with the meaning of care as part of paid work; and its problematic character is at the heart of nursing debates, whether concerned with professional status, the conflict between holism and specialism, the character of the knowledge base, struggles with doctors. Of all occupations, nursing bears most clearly the marks of its origins in assumptions about gender, and in this final section we will review some of the ways nursing theorists have conceptualised this relationship and its relevance to debates about carework generally.

Davies (1995) approaches nursing through a conscious focus on gender rather than women; she makes a clear distinction between concrete men and women and cultural codes or representations of gender, in the form of masculinity and femininity. This allows her to show how jobs are gendered, separate from the sex of individuals who occupy them. As Acker (1990) argues, organisations are not just neutral frameworks into which people of male or female gender are fitted unequally, but are themselves gendered. The job slots into which individuals fit are shaped by the processes of gender in such a way that those at the top of the organisation are formed around the attributes of masculinity and many of those at the bottom around the attributes of femininity. Not all women occupy female jobs. Some, particularly those with professional status (female doctors, women vice chancellors), operate with a bifurcated vision in which major aspects of their working lives are structured according to masculine principles. Others occupy jobs, like nurses or careworkers, whose nature is profoundly shaped by principles of femininity. This remains so, even when such jobs are undertaken by men; though as we saw in Chapter 6, the consequences of such cross-gender work are different for men and women.

Focusing on masculinity and femininity has, of course, its dangers, threatening to freeze stereotypes of sexual difference; and emphasising difference has traditionally been used in conservative discourse to perpetuate male dominance and disqualify women from areas of work or public life where the rewards are high. This problem can be met, however, by emphasising the plural and historically contingent nature of the differences – masculini*ties* and feminini*ties* – and by acknowledging the dimension of power whereby cultural representations of gender systematically privilege masculinity (Davies 1995).

This privileging extends to the concepts of social science themselves, as Bologh argues in her reinterpretation of Weber's bureaucratic rationality. For Weber, the public sphere is an implicitly masculine one of hostile strangers in which individual men compete for and strive after power and domination, albeit at times mediated by the pursuit of certain non-instrumental values. This vision creates a cold, harsh world in which the values and practices of 'caring' have no part. Emotions, enthusiasms, vulnerabilities and commitments get in the way of its logic; rather they belong to the world of women and of home. Femininity represents the reverse of these public values, and as such can only be cultivated and protected if it is withdrawn into the private sphere. Women here become confined to the life of home, and in classic Victorian accounts become like unrepressed children, lively, sweet, emotional, sympathetic, relying on the guidance of their feelings rather than abstract rationality. Femininity, for these Weberian men, is feared as a temptation, something that is seductive but contemptible, and that must therefore be repressed in themselves, rigorously confined to the private sphere and the persons of women. Caring both at home and in the workplace is caught in this matrix of repression and fear (Davies 1998).

This account in terms of the emergence of bourgeois concepts of masculinity and femininity and the related separation of public and private spheres is used by Davies to explain what happens when the values of the private sphere in the form of caring are transferred across into the world of work; for the denial of and repression of the principles that femininity stands for, operate not just in the division of public and private spheres, but within the public sphere also. The public world and its language is defined by the vision of masculinity. In entering this world, women are called to either – like female doctors – renounce their female cultural identity or – as with nurses – find themselves defined as female; silenced, neglected and misunderstood if they try to articulate and uphold values that do not fit with instrumental action. Nursing is caught between the dominant – and masculine – discourses of health care: the positivistic science of medicine and the economic rationality of managerialism (Lawler 1997).

As Reverby (1987) showed in her historical account of the emergence of hospital nursing out of the home, nurses are called to care in a culture that does not value caring. They are expected to uphold values of female identity in the face of a masculinity that is profoundly ambivalent about it, and in the face of institutions imbued with such masculinity. Dunlop (1986) similarly argues that 'caring' work emerges as a response to people-work as it moved out of the private domain into the public world of health care. Women workers were required to humanise the system through their caring work in these new service occupations. Nursing thus took on the problematic role of translating 'love' into the public domain. But in doing so, this work has kept some of its private nature. Like bodywork more generally, nursing is perceived as something that is done in a context that is intimate and private. When transferred to the public sphere it retains these associations, and they reinforce the tendency for caring to be hidden, unacknowledged work.

Carework is also hidden because of its relationship with masculine concepts of work. As Acker (1990) and others have argued the concept of a 'job' is itself gendered, resting as it does on assumptions about workers that derive from male norms: ones that prioritise full-time work, permit long hours and assume a particular organisation of domestic life in which men's primary needs for intimacy and closeness are met in the family and in the persons of their wives. Formal accounts of organisations rest on masculinist logic that subdivides and ranks tasks, and ignores activities that do not fit into its matrixes. The public world is thus made to appear rational, orderly and controlled. But many of the tasks performed by women workers do not fit into this. Carework, as we have seen, is particularly hard to capture in this way; job analyses, with their minute task divisions, often fail to recognise its character, and trivialise its complexity (Neysmith and Aronson 1996).

This public world of rationality also contains its own instabilities. It is difficult to inhabit: inflexible, cold and does not meet all the needs that arise in organisations. As a result, special categories of gendered occupations – like secretaries and nurses – have emerged to deal with these difficulties. The rational bureaucracy is thus 'supported' by the gendered work of secretaries. These office wives work in a flexible, individual and informal way, attending to the emotional and personal needs of male bosses. It is because secretaries do this emotional labour – that is unconceptualised, devalued and ignored – that bosses can continue to present their work in terms of the abstract rational ideal. Masculine rationality tries to drive out the feminine but cannot exist without it (Pringle 1989).

In a parallel way nursing makes possible the masculine activity of medicine. The medical encounter is fleeting and formalised and rests on the suppression of emotion on both sides. But it is only made possible by the preparatory and supportive work of nurses who record the patients' data, smooth the encounter, tidy up after the doctor has left and deliver the prescribed regime. Nursing is not a profession, Davies argues, so much as an adjunct to a concept of profession, that is itself gendered. Part of the definition of nursing work is what medicine rejects or fails to see. This underwrites its unbounded and undefined character. It represents *all the rest*. Like women themselves it is constructed as the Other to the profession of medicine. From this perspective the earlier feminist project of making care visible was simplistic:

It is not that caring has somehow been overlooked, and can be retrieved and added to a pre-existing framework. It is rather that the denial of caring is central to the construction of the public world. Bringing in caring means unmasking the binary gendered thought that bolsters masculinity.

(Davies 1998: 135)

Conclusion

Carework is typically analysed in terms of the debate on care as it emerged out of the analysis of family caregiving. But, as we have seen in the last two chapters, such a focus is not always the most helpful way in which to analyse the sector. Family-based care, although it shares many common features with carework, is quite distinct and follows its own logic, and it cannot be understood separately from the structures of kinship and long-term family obligation. Carework by contrast is premised on a different set of relations, albeit ones that at times draw on familial models. Avoiding the links with informal care and analysing it primarily as a form of paid labour also helps us to demystify 'care'. These are jobs that are shaped by similar forces to those structuring other forms of paid employment. As such, carework needs to be set on the context of other paid occupations, particularly those in the service and health care sectors. They too have a strongly gendered character. The clearest parallels are with nursing, which also unites bodywork elements with emotional and nurturant ones; and nursing has similarly struggled to establish space for the recognition of the care element in its activities, against accounts that have trivialised, downplayed and rendered such work invisible. In nursing's case the struggle has taken place in the context of tensions around relations with medicine, though latterly also with managerialism. With carework the conflict is less overt, though many of the same themes occur. Carework is, like nursing, constructed around a gendered concept of labour in which its main activities are naturalised in the persons of women. Both have traditionally rested on a concept of the 'good woman'. Nightingale's nurses were famously 'good women' (though they were much more as well). And as we have seen, careworkers self-identify with being caring persons, and indeed are perceived to be such by employers also, though such a recognition does not translate into the formal work contact. Rather it is contained within the implicit gender contract.

The emotional labour of care is also closely linked to the gendered character of the work (though as we noted in Chapter 6, men who do this work also experience the job in terms of emotional labour). There is an unbounded element in carework that derives from the importation into it of an ethic of love that derives from the primary bonds of the family. This is something that workers find it hard to resist and they find themselves caught between the personalised demands of this ethic of care – reinforced by the emotional bonds that develop over time, particularly in response to personal dependence – and the conditions of wage labour in an increasingly hard-nosed and cost-pressured sector.

Carework needs therefore to be conceptualised as part of a much wider sociological issue concerning the nature of social action in the public sphere and the problematic character of the traditional analysis of this that itself arose out of the historically contingent emergence of the modern world. In this, care – like the body – has been relegated to a hidden, unacknowledged category of action and one that sociology is only just beginning to address.

9 The power dynamics of care

Domiciliary care is a site of conflict in which two social groups, both of whom suffer from a wider social diminishment, struggle to establish autonomy and personal esteem. Clients struggle to resist the domination of workers and to maintain a fragile sense of self in the face of the erosions of disability and age. Workers strive to establish control over their work and to extract from it sources of esteem and status. Although these conflicting aims are played out in the confined space of the home and the close intimacies of body care, they reflect larger tensions deriving from the wider society concerning class, 'race', age and gender. In this chapter we will explore the nature of these power struggles as experienced in the care encounter, focusing in particular on 'race' and class. But before doing so we need to look at some of the general features of bathing and body work that underlie these dynamics, for the power struggles of care are far from equal and are heavily weighted in favour of the workers.

Power and domination

To discuss power in the context of the body inevitably raises the influence of Foucault. Though this is not a Foucauldian study as such, bathing contains a number of strongly Foucauldian themes. The body for Foucault is the prime site for the exercise of power; and his work has alerted us to the complex ways in which power operates on and through the body. Power for Foucault is all around and in and through us. It operates at a covert and micro level, flowing through the minutest parts of the social system, and is constitutive of it. Disciplinary practices are the means whereby the principles of carcereal society are institutionalised in everyday routines. Foucault thus addresses precisely the areas of the mundane, the ordinary and the bodily that are the focus of this study, showing how these provide the setting for the exercise of power and domination.

Social welfare systems are part of this. This is easiest to see in relation to professionals like doctors, social workers, psychologists who through their practices, and the discourses that relate to them, exercise disciplinary power on a day-to-day basis. However, lower level workers like care assistants in residential homes, auxiliaries on long-stay wards, and careworkers in private homes also exercise disciplinary power, ordering and managing bodies, and their role parallels that of the wardens in prisons and nurses in asylums analysed by Foucault.

As we saw in Chapter 2, running through the history and practice of bathing is a dark, coercive strain. This arises most clearly where people *are* bathed, where their bodies are exposed, directed and made subject to the control and will of another, rendered, in Foucault's terms, docile. We saw how baths frequently feature as rites of passage into the institution whereby individuals are stripped of their social identity and made subject to the regime. We also saw how baths have featured as part of coercive techniques in relation to medicine, psychiatry and penology, and how these aspects become all the stronger when mediated by machinery which acts to distance and objectify the bodies, at the same time as trapping and caging them. By and large these powerful sadistic themes are not directly in play in relation to domiciliary bathing, and the tone is a gentler, less coercive one. However they form part of the background noise of care, and we have heard echoes of them earlier in relation to bathing equipment in institutions and day centres, as well as the masks, aprons and gloves of workers.

The power dynamics of bathing are inherently unequal. One person, strong and able, stands above and over another who is frail and physically vulnerable, forced to rely on their strength and good will. The client is stripped of their clothes, while the bathing attendant retains theirs. Being naked in the face of someone who is not, contains a powerful dynamic of domination and vulnerability, and it is often used in situations of interrogation or torture as a means of subjugating the individual. The dynamic of nakedness is thus one in which the client is the structurally weaker and more vulnerable party. Receiving help with bathing also requires the client to offer themselves up as a object for surveillance. Their bodies are made subject to the gaze of a worker, part of whose task may be to evaluate and monitor their state. Community nurses traditionally valued bathing as a means of reviewing the state of the patient's body; and although such interventions are benign in intent, they reinforce the dynamic of surveillance and observation. Furthermore, as we saw in Chapter 3, many older people have internalised a view that their bodies are unpleasant, and that looking at or touching them is distasteful. Aging within modern western culture is in part perceived as a form of failure, and exposing your body for judgement, particularly by a younger person, is often experienced as a form of diminishment.

There is in addition a powerful dynamic in western culture, whereby to be reduced to, or pointedly associated with, the body is to be denigrated and diminished. We saw how for disabled people, particularly disabled women, being reduced to their bodies was a particularly demeaning form of treatment, one that eroded the self and presented the individual as an object to be viewed – a body rather than a person. In a similar way, women in sexist culture are described in terms of their bodies, or parts of their bodies, made subject to the male phallic gaze. Even the widespread avoidance of direct bodily description of individuals in polite conversation reflects something of this sense that to emphasise the body of a person is in some way to lessen them.

It is this sense that partly underlies the unease that many including myself have felt over applying the Foucauldian model – the sense that Foucault's emphasis on bodies represents something that is of itself oppressive, a process in which people are rendered as objects, silenced, dominated, exposed to public gaze by the nature of the analysis itself. I have explored this issue more fully elsewhere (Twigg 2000); the problem turns around the sense that in such accounts the research materials – individuals in the study – are made subject to an essentially sadistic analysis, in which author and reader together conspire to dominate and render them docile. Recasting the focus of the analysis in terms of bodies rather than people, as Foucauldian accounts tend to do, is inevitably a form of diminishment and a denial of subjectivity. Part of the Foucauldian project, of course, is precisely to destabilise the Enlightenment concept of the subject, but this poses difficulties for any study – as this does – that attempts to give weight to the subjective accounts of users. It is not by chance that Foucauldian accounts nearly always present the social world from the outside, from a distant, all-seeing perspective that conspires in the processes that it describes, and that rarely attempts to encompass a plurality of viewpoints; for example few Foucauldian accounts of the disciplinary work of doctors, nurses or careworkers attempt to include the views and responses of clients. The difficulty is felt most strongly at the experiential, reflexive level of doing the research where there is an inevitable unease at applying such an analysis to the vulnerable but vividly present people with whom one is interacting in the interview, though it applies as much to the conceptual level of presenting the analysis.

These difficulties have their roots in two of the classic criticisms of Foucault: that his account denies human agency, and that is it is overly pre-occupied with issues of order and control. As Wilson (2000) argues, the bodies it deals in are 'complaisant', subordinated; and the embodied individual is seen primarily as a site for the investigation of social order, rather than a source of human agency. Under a Foucauldian approach, the whole intellectual enterprise of the sociology of the body is made subordinate to the question of social order. But such an approach limits the scope of the analysis, telling us little of the ways in which individuals' experience the world from their perspectives; and in a study of this kind that is a major conceptual drawback.

Equality and power

Emphasising the body can, in certain circumstances, be a marker of equality and intimacy. At various points, we have noted how bodily closeness contains the capacity to create intimacy, though in the context of the care encounter an intimacy that is not always welcome and that sometimes contains ambivalent elements. Similarly, shared bodily processes can underwrite equality. We saw how careworkers at times attempt to resist this equality, putting up barriers between themselves and close contact with clients, for example by restricting the implied equality of shared meals to favoured clients only. Before the body we are all equal. There is a commonplace saying that even the Queen goes to the toilet; and the phrase is usually deployed as a robust assertion of equality and denial that people with power or status are any different from us fundamentally. Psychological empowerment techniques for dealing with powerful and dominating people sometimes use this dynamic, encouraging the individual to visualise the frightening person sitting on the lavatory. To be viewed in such a position is, of course, about more than just an assertion of the equality of the body. It is a technique of denigration. As we shall see, some careworkers are aware of the power that such bodily exposure of clients gives to them, and in situations of conflict use it to bolster their esteem. Here bodily exposure is one-way and asymmetrical, used to underwrite relations of domination.

An account in terms of power, domination and the creation of docile bodies is not, however, the whole story. Bathing is a site of conflict and struggle in which the dynamics of power are not wholly one way. The recipients of care do have some resources to deploy in the exchange. Some of these derive from the ideology of public provision. The official account of social services is not one of docile bodies and disciplined clients; and indeed such language is abhorrent to the social-work values that inform social services and which, in theory at least, aim to support and empower older people. Though care services often fail to live up to these ideals, it is important not to overlook their role. Values of empowerment and of care are widely endorsed within social services, and attempts are made to promote them at the front line. The official job description of carework is to provide a sensitive, caring service that respects the autonomy of the client; and workers are in some degree constrained in their relations with clients by such definitions. 'Being caring' is officially part of the job. Although workers internalise this ethic to varying degrees, most who stay in the sector endorse its values. Managers also make efforts to weed out careworkers who have the wrong attitude. The context of provision is thus one which endorses the wishes of clients, to some degree at least.

These official definitions of the work are reinforced by the emotional dynamics of carework. As we have seen, close contact over time creates a sense of fellow feeling and concern. Careworkers often develop strong emotional bonds with clients, particularly with those who are heavily dependent on them – those who in the conventional sense are the least powerful – so that dependence creates its own form of power, acting in part to redress the balance, or at least to impose internalised constraints upon the full exercise of power by workers.

Lastly clients have resources that derive from wider structures of society. As we saw in Chapter 4, the fact that domiciliary care takes place in the homes of recipients endows them with a degree of power; and the commonly shared ideology of home constrains the degree to which workers can act freely. The limited period of time in which workers are in the house also puts limits on the extent of their potential domination of the client. This is in marked contrast to the situation in the residential home. The power dynamics of care are also mediated by structures of 'race' and class, and these can endow certain clients at least, with an element of power in the exchange.

The struggle for control

Domestic cleaning was a prime area of conflict for many older and disabled clients. The quality of their home surroundings was important to them and they found not being able to control and maintain them frustrating and depressing – a finding reflected in other studies (Walker and Warren 1996, Neysmith and Aronson 1996). Many struggled to get the work done to their satisfaction. They mainly attributed the problem to the poor domestic skills of the younger generation, explaining resignedly that they just did not know how to clean; but they felt that their attitude was poor, lackadaisical and more a matter of show than substance. 'Most of them are what I call theatre dusters', commented Mrs Elster tartly, 'they flick instead of wiping up.' These were not class-based attitudes; and comments about the poor quality of the work were expressed at all social levels, indeed some of the strongest criticism came from working-class women who had prided themselves on the state of their homes. These expectations pose problems for agencies since no provision, whether in the public or commercial sector, can meet the standards maintained by some individuals for themselves by choice. Many authorities also limit the domestic tasks that they are willing to cover, excluding high dusting, paintwork and windows; and some, as we saw in Chapter 5, have withdrawn from the area of cleaning altogether, leaving it to private provision.

It was clear, however, that clients were often not making impossibly high demands so much as experiencing difficulty in getting careworkers to do the tasks that were a standard part of their job description but that they disliked or regarded as beneath them. This was particularly an issue in London where the home care service had difficulty in recruiting, and relied heavily on agency staff. Joshua who worked for the voluntary service bathing service described how many clients:

> are scared of telling the home help that, can you empty the bin or wash the things in the sink or so you know. They are scared to say ... Some of them they don't like the home helps because of the way the home helps do to them, like they don't come on regular times. When they come they are very strict, if you give them a lot to do, they'll say 'Oh no I'm not going to finish all this you know.'

In London some home helps appear to pick and choose what tasks they will undertake, and these tend to be the lighter more attractive ones. Washing the kitchen floor and cleaning the toilet are not among these. Some clients are afraid to challenge the workers. Mrs Ostrovski felt that that home care workers – some of whom she described as wives of foreign PhD students – were too superior to do this mundane work and she hired a Polish women to clean the loo. Descibing some Somali workers she declared:

> I never ask them to do anything for me. I even don't ask them to take the rubbish out. I just tell them to post things, or go to the shop and buy me a Coca Cola or something like that. And I said to [the home care organiser], 'For God's sake, can't you send somebody who is.' I mean, I haven't got the nerve – you have this beautiful woman you know, nearly two metres … How can I tell her she's supposed to go and wash my bathroom and my loo? … I mean. [pauses] They are not cleaners.

While I was in the flat the careworker did arrive, dressed in a white lace blouse and skirt, garments that gave a very clear message about the limits of the kind of work she was willing to do.

In Mrs Elster's case the battle for control was direct and open. She felt that workers disliked being told what to do and were very touchy if corrected:

> You've got to handle with gloves, velvet gloves, because they get to very uptight about things especially when it's their fault. They don't like it, being told, although I try and do it as nicely as I can…. They're very touchy.

She found it difficult to cope with workers who grumbled, were resentful and did not get on with the work:

> A few years back now a girl came, she was only about 18 or 20 and it was a very cold winter, one of our icy winters, and she's got sandals on, no stockings and a little short skirt up here and she was going around, 'Oh it's so cold in here! It's so cold in here!' So I said to her, 'Forgive me for suggesting it, but why don't you have some shoes or stockings on.'

Mrs Elster had been a vendeuse in a couturier house, and although confined to bed retained a certain elegance with her black hair drawn back in a bun, her earrings and vivid make up. The tone of the quotation conveys something of the antagonism that can arise from combined differences of age and class.

In general, clients dislike having to tell workers what to do. This is partly because it seems to make the relationship like that of a servant, which is something that many feel uneasy about. Giving instructions was also exhausting. As Mrs Forsyth explained 'when you're in pain, you really haven't got the energy to start telling them'; and the sense of having constantly to explain everything was one of the reasons why frequent changes of careworker were particularly disliked. Being explicit about the body was also something people felt uncomfortable about. These are areas that are traditionally managed by avoiding direct speech; having to articulate needs in relation to them was embarrassing. What people wanted was the perfect careworker who anticipated their needs and did what was wanted without having to be asked. As Mrs Kennelly, a working class widow, explained, her best worker:

> sees what has to be done. You don't have to ask her. Like she see the clothes horse, with all clothes on it drying. She'll feel them, get them off, fold them and put them away. Now don't get me wrong, the other girls, if I ask them, would you empty the clothes horse, they say yes. They'll do anything, *but I've got to tell them*. That's the difference. One will automatically do it.

It is a fine line, however, between anticipating wishes and taking over. Clients may not want to direct the workers actively, but they do want to retain their independence and not to fall under the control of the worker. A manager in Coastville had been concerned by some quality assurance work which they had commissioned in which a number of their workers were described by clients as 'bossy'. In the study, some clients described conflicts with careworkers who were domineering. Mrs Colegate, a middle aged woman with MS, described such workers:

MRS COLEGATE: They were very loud, very loud and um, tend to take over when they got into the house and I'm afraid I don't like people like that.
INTERVIEWER: How did they take over?
MRS COLEGATE: Bit bombastic, well sort of, I'm in charge and you've gotta do what I say.

Sharon Kimpton, a working-class women in her thirties with muscle disease, recounted one particularly bad experience with a careworker who was overbearing and talked down to her:

She used to make me feel small.... that was the sort of person she was.... If you had views, you know, her views were stronger than yours ... Like I was a young kid.

This was particularly unpleasant in the bath where the worker's dominance took the form of reducing Sharon to a baby: 'She was like mothering me ... like I was still a little baby and, you know, cuddling me, getting me out the bath.'

This was a relationship that Sharon did not want, and felt was being imposed on her. She was being required to accept a form of infantalisation as the price of getting help, and 'care' here went far beyond what was wanted or needed:

SHARON: She insisted on bathing me as well, so she washed me everywhere with gloves on.
INTERVIEWER: What, she washed your private parts and—
SHARON: Yeah, yeah.
INTERVIEWER   Bottom and everything?
SHARON :   Yeah.
SHARON'S MOTHER: Oh, she was really bossy, wasn't she?
SHARON: Yeah, I told you she was. I told her, you know: 'You don't have to stay, you can do the bedrooms if you want,' and she went: 'Oh no, no, no, I'll make sure you're alright.'

Lee-Treweek (1996) argues that in the power struggles of care, clients are often required to accept emotional infantalisation as part of the price of receiving help. Residents in the care home were obliged to enter into relationships in which they were treated as sweet little children, showing weakness, receiving hugs, displaying gratitude. Any resistance produced coldness from the workers and the withdrawal of human contact. The one group of residents in the home that workers really resented were those that maintained their distance and treated the place like a hotel. This was unpardonable because it denied workers their emotional dominance and reward, placing them in the position of a servant.

Complaining is difficult because the relationship is so personal. As Mrs Gray explained in relation to a worker who rushed the bath 'I didn't say it to her because she's very nice, I didn't like to upset her.' Complaining also creates a bad feeling that can be awkward, given the close interpersonal nature of the work. This is particularly the case when the careworker is the client's only companion. Sharing long periods of time with someone with whom one is on bad terms is unpleasant and stressful, as Mrs Elster found. 'I need somebody, like anybody in my position, who's fairly efficient, and is cheerfullish cos I'm miserable enough on my own, without having somebody grizzling, grumbling.' If client and worker are not getting on, things become very claustrophobic. It is the intimacy of the situation that makes the struggle for power so direct and so highly charged.

Careworkers also engage in the struggle for dominance. At the simplest level they need to exert control over the conditions of their work. Often this is difficult as the surroundings are not theirs, and rarely well adapted to the task. At some level at least, they are 'guests' in the house. Also as Lee-Treweek (1998) points out in relation to residential care, the materials they work with – the bodies of the old – can prove recalcitrant and difficult to manage. Workers also need to establish control over the time element in the work. Carework is increasingly monitored in terms of time, and in order to get the work done and off to the next appointment, workers need to impose a certain pace on the activity and to control and limit the exchange. As Desiree explained:'if they're having a bath if they want to relax, I don't mind that. But then I sometimes put a restriction on the length of time that they um, relax for.' Disciplining clients in the sense of making them conform to time discipline and other forms of ordering and control is a central element in the work.

Reluctant bathers pose particular problems. Careworkers felt that that it was their duty to impose certain standards of hygiene. As Desiree explained, if she felt a person should have a bath, she would give it, pretty well regardless. Describing one client she explained:

DESIREE: I always think it's important that they have a bath every day, or at least when they can....
INTERVIEWER: Has she asked you to help that way?
DESIREE: No, I just thought she needed to have a bath. As I said, she just, she doesn't have a bath and she won't, because she hasn't got the memory to have a bath.

Another London worker described how clients sometimes tried to avoid a bath and had to be hunted down:

DAWN: They are crafty though, because Mr. Smith ... he lives in a block of flats where there's a bar, opens at three o'clock, and I go to bath him at half past three and he's missing and he's hiding up in the corner of the bar.
TONI: Yes, a lot of them are like that.

DAWN: Doesn't want to have his bath. He said 'This is all too much for me,' he said.

Avoidance is particularly a problem with people with dementia who often cease to bother about personal hygiene and resent the disturbance and intrusion that dealing with it entails. Bathing and washing are thus common areas of struggle and difficulty for careworkers, particularly where they are officially rostered to do such work as part of the care plan. As a result many developed techniques of persuasion that at times border on the coercive in order to get the job done.

Careworkers dislike being closely ordered and controlled. We saw this in Mrs Elster's account, and her perception was endorsed by the careworkers. Clients with, what were termed 'exacting rituals', were seen as particularly tiresome:

> One lady I was doing and she had all these buckets and stuff in her shower. I took them all out, and then when I put them all in again, I put them back, I tried to remember where, cos I was told she was very particular, and I put this bucket back, and she was like, no, no two inches to the left and one inch to the right, that's how particular she was.

Such close control and overt direction were seen as beyond the acceptable, turning the worker into a servant.

Rejecting the status of a servant

Rejecting the status of a servant lies at the heart of the power struggle of care. It is this model of the relationship that careworkers are at pains to resist. The reasons for this lie in the history of class relations and the related development of work identities as they developed into the modern era. To be a servant is to be personally subordinated to another, and as such it is fundamentally at odds with the core values of personal autonomy and individualism that mark modern western society. Gregson and Lowe (1994) quote Coser in describing being a servant as typical of pre-modern work: no defined hours, no formal limits to the work, based on personal affiliation, with expectations of loyalty. It is the directly personal nature of the subordination that is significant here. Many modern jobs involve subordination. What is particular about being a servant is its personal character, servicing the needs and wishes of another. That is what is deeply resented; and that is what the careworkers seek to avoid.

The history of domestic service is central in the formation of class and gender relations. During the nineteenth and early twentieth centuries, domestic service formed the largest source of employment for women. Middle and upper-class women were able to live relatively leisured lives as a result of employing, mainly female, servants. As a result, one in four women employed in 1851 was in domestic service (Burnett 1974). The sector went into rapid decline after the First World War when the expansion of manufacturing and office-based work enabled women to pursue alternative sources of employment that offered the freedom of a more contract-based relationship in which they were not required to be personally subordinated and in which home and workspace were separated. This flight of women from domestic service had important consequences for class and gender relations. During the post-Second-World-War era, a new equality in class – though not gender – terms was imposed, in that domestic labour came to be performed by *both* middle and working-class women. (Gendered inequality for some women increased, in that middle and upper-class women now performed domestic labour directly for their husbands.) These changes created a fundamental shift in the experience of class relations among women, in that middle- and working-class women were no longer directly engaged in employer/employee relations.

The trend away from domestic service was reinforced in the post-war era by the general shift towards a self-servicing economy in which people substituted material goods for personal service (Gershuny 1978). Not all forms of domestic labour are, however, capable of being mediated by new technology, and domestic cleaning remains relatively labour intensive and linked to the setting of the home. From the 1980s onwards there has been a minor reversal of the overall trend, with the growth of domestic cleaning work in middle-class homes. The new employers are typically married women who use class-, and to some degree race-, inequalities to mitigate against their own gendered disadvantage in marriage (Gregson and Lowe 1994).

These changes affect the experience of home care, for they provide the backdrop against which activities like cleaning are evaluated, and they explain why attempts by clients to reassert relations of personal service are resented and resisted by the workers. Careworkers are in general at pains to emphasise their status as carers and not cleaners. Cleaning work is clearly identified as demeaning when compared with care. These class-based feelings are not confined to Britain, but are found in North American and Scandinavian work too (Waerness 1987, Neysmith and Aronson 1997). There is a 'race' dimension also. In the USA, cleaning work has historically been associated with black women. As Neysmith and Aronson found, where care tasks were done by women of color in private homes, elderly clients and their families often responded to them as if they were domestic servants. A number of studies have reported how black workers resented being termed the 'maid' and would sometimes quit the job rather than being made subject to such assumptions (Neysmith and Aronson 1997, Eustis *et al* 1993, Diamond 1992).

Careworkers in general prefer to present their work in terms of caring, and not cleaning. Though the majority in the study were contracted to do both personal care and housework, most disliked the cleaning element and if possible avoided it, regarding it as of lower status: 'I don't like to be classed [as] a home help. I'm a carer, and I don't do housework or the dusting, and I don't wanna be called the home help.'

Warren similarly found that support workers in an innovative community care scheme resented being seen as cleaners or skivvys, or even worse 'scrubbers' by the clients (Warren 1994).

Careworkers felt that clients had less respect for them if they did cleaning as well as care: 'These people, once you go there to do the clean, they don't want to know whom you are ... they don't believe we are carer, they believe we cleaner.'

When they did personal care, clients sometimes mistook them for nurses, and some careworkers were gratified to be spoken to in that way: 'They say "Nurse", they actually call you "Nurse". But then when you're shopping for them or owt like that, it's "Pat".'

Emphasising the care element in the work has an obvious appeal in placing it nearer the professional model of nursing. As Desiree explained:

> I like the personal care. I like to be involved a bit more than just being the cleaner ... You just feel more professional ... And a lot of the clients they ... they think we're more better than the district nurses (laughing).

Emphasising caring was a claim for semi-professional status, and those careworkers like Desiree who were keen for personal advancement, wanted to present the work in those terms. Desiree was one of the few workers who favoured uniforms, and saw them as a means of upgrading and smartening the work.

But caring is also viewed as better because it avoids the demeaning connotations of being a servant, someone at the personal behest of another, having to clean their lavatory and kneel and scrub their carpet.

LENORE: Socially, you know caring is a bit neater than cleaning.
INTERVIEWER: A bit neater?
LENORE: Yes.
INTERVIEWER: Meaning?
LENORE: Meaning when you go to someone's place and you have to do the toilet, to do the bath, but 'care' you deal with only the hygiene ...
JESSIE: Yes, the personal hygiene.
LENORE: True there is some dirty aspect of it but as a woman you know you don't bother ... I prefer that side than go, some of you, some of them will be asking you to be scrubbing their carpet that there are spots there, you have to bend down scrubbing.

As we shall see with Mrs Elster, the whole issue of bodily demeanour, bending and kneeling, was a highly charged one, particularly in the context of 'race'.

Care is also preferred because the personal dynamics of care are more equal. The cleaner is a distant person, working under orders. When the care is intimate and close, however, it is harder for the client to maintain psychological distance and control. As a result careworkers can establish their dominance in the hands-on work of intimate care in a way that they cannot when just cleaning the house. Becoming a carer therefore means gaining a capacity to control, and with that some status, in the context of a job that has relatively little in the eyes of the wider employment world.

The body element here operates in an ambivalent way. In some senses doing things of an intimate nature in conditions of servitude might seem more demeaning, approaching the status of the body servant, subjugated in the directly bodily way that we referred to in the chapter on the nature of bodywork. But in other ways, it offers opportunities for the assertion of equality and for a reversal of status. Intimate body care offers the chance to exert Foucauldian bio-power. As we have seen, the dynamics of body care – the asymmetrical nakedness, the bodily posture, the exposure of the person in situations that are normally hidden – all reinforce the power of the worker and enable her to establish dominance in the exchange.

These struggles for power and dominance in care raise questions that have been discussed within the disability movement, in particular in relation to the ideal of personal assistance. The model of the personal assistant developed out of the anger and frustration of disabled people at being under the thumb of professionals. Professionals, disability activists argued, have chosen to spend large sums of money developing services that control disabled people rather than allowing them to control their own lives. Gaining control over this money through the medium of direct payments (initially in Britain through the Disabled Living Fund, but from 1993 directly through Direct Payments) and being able to use it to hire and fire personal assistants was an important step in the fight to achieve autonomy (Morris 1993, 1997, Kestenbaum 1996).

The ideal of the personal assistant is that the worker should act like the arms and legs of the disabled person, doing their bidding in an exact and neutral way, requiring no special explanations or gratitude, simply following instructions. This is quite distinct from 'being cared for' in the traditional way, in which the worker is the active agent doing the caring and the disabled person is a passive recipient of attention. At its extreme, the ideal of the personal assistant can seem to imply a denial of the personhood of the worker who is required to efface him or herself totally. It certainly approaches near to the model of the servant that careworkers are at pains to resist. One manager in the study described her concern in taking over responsibility for a personal assistant situation to find that her staff member was expected to sit in the back bedroom when not needed, to be summoned by a bell when required. The manager felt that this was quite unacceptable, and she had supported workers in refusing to operate on this basis. The bell, with its resonances of maids and servants, was clearly critical in defining the unacceptable nature of the relationship.

Though the rhetoric of personal assistance emphasises the wholly neutral nature of the relationship in which the personal assistant is under the command of the client, the reality is never that simple. It is impossible to eradicate interpersonal aspects from the exchange; and indeed disabled users are themselves ambivalent about attempts to do so, uncertain how far totally neutral relations are desirable or possible. It is also very difficult to get workers to abandon ideas of responsibility that rest on professional models of care and are at odds with the logic of consumerist control (Ungerson 1999). Carers want to retain a sense of themselves as professionally in charge. Conflict is endemic in such relations; Eustis and her colleagues (1994) found power struggles featured in about one third of the client–worker relations they studied.

Personal assistants are often life stage workers, young and with as yet no family commitments; and they are doing the work as a prelude to something else. The total quality of the response can be something that appeals to the idealism of the young when they are not so firmly located in the social structures of status and class. This can protect the self identity and esteem of such workers, enabling them to be more self-effacing, more able to put the wishes of another first. They are able to give in a total way because they know they are going to move on in their lives. This response was particularly characteristic of workers in the voluntary sector bathing scheme, many of whom were transitional workers. The scheme, in the view of clients, local social services managers and the researcher, gave a particularly high quality service. In addition, the workers had the advantage that they specialised in bathing work and were not involved in the menial activity of cleaning, and were thus protected from the erosion of status that that implied. But for the other workers in home care or private agencies, the struggle for esteem was more direct. Letting oneself become subordinate in order to allow the client to take control of the encounter could be personally undermining, and it threatened the fragile esteem surrounding the work. For these workers, whose labour market choices were often constrained, putting oneself consciously below the clients, so as to allow them to take charge, had limited appeal.

'Race'

The power dynamics of care are mediated through the intersecting structures of 'race' and class. 'Race' as an issue in community care has largely been analysed in terms of the disadvantaged position of black ethnic minority people in service receipt; and a number of studies have charted the structural barriers black ethnic minority users and carers face in the form of: inappropriate and inaccessible services; partial and inadequate understanding of their needs and views; assumptions about cultural practices; and the racist attitudes of service providers (Ahmad and Atkin 1996, Law 1996). Such writers have pointed to the dualist experience of black ethnic minority people in social services, under-represented in relation to the more advantageous forms of social care, such as sheltered housing, home help, day care, but over-represented in relation to the social control functions of social services such as admissions to psychiatric hospitals, detention centres or compulsory admission of children to care. Dominelli (1992) argues that this dualism receives a further reinforcement through the predominant location of black ethnic minority social workers in those sectors of social services that are regarded as less desirable and at the sharp end of social work practice where they are more directly engaged in controlling people's behaviour. Her comments mainly relate to social work, but they apply also to the carework sector in general where black ethnic minority people are more often employed in areas like mental disability or psychogeriatrics where they are required to control and discipline clients. Black ethnic minority workers are thus differentially positioned in the harsher and more punitive parts of the welfare system dealing with the least powerful clients.

Within the bathing study, issues around 'race' – and class – were most marked in the London sample where the majority of the careworkers were of black or ethnic minority working-class background, and most of the clients white, of mixed social background. Among the clients there was a range of responses to this. Some expressed fairly straightforwardly racist views. We have already noted how in western culture direct reference to the body is one of the ways of denigrating or reducing the status of a person, and these comments took the classic racist form of bodily references focusing on toilet habits and smells (Largey and Watson 1972). Mrs Fitzgerald, commenting on how she missed her earlier white careworker with whom she got on so well, explained how it was different with black workers:

> Partly language, and also – I may be wrong here, but I think most white people, we have similar toilet habits – they may have quite different ones – I don't know, I don't know anything about that, because I never discuss it with them ... I'm not really anti these people, I just rather wish they weren't here because the country is so small and we're getting so crowded, and they seem to be overcrowding us.

Later, commenting on an unsatisfactory worker who had been sent to do her shopping, she explained:

> She shopped for herself and then bought my stuff and then she came back here, and on top of all that, she smelt. So I stopped it.... She was black, but her clothes were spotless and she was one of those unfortunate people that suffer that way, but it was

unbearable, and to think my food had been carried by it – oh, I didn't want it.

Most evinced more mixed views. They identified 'race' as an issue, but at the same time recognised that individual black careworkers were very good and caring. 'Race' was available as a category, as it were lying around, waiting to be deployed as a form of explanation when things went wrong. Miss Henderson for example praised her special careworker – 'I've got Susie who's a darling person'– who was black, but at the same time felt that black careworkers were often rough and uncaring, belligerent and rude:

MISS HENDERSON: I'm sorry I have to say, I'm not anti-racial at all but some of these black girls are very arrogant and belligerent and rude. Very brisk anyhow.... I think it's because they've got a chip on their shoulder, they are like this. But I've noticed it, quite a lot of the agency people who are black are much less caring.
INTERVIEWER: In what sort of ways?
MISS HENDERSON: Well, as I say, the attitude of, the attitude of doing anything for you. It's a chore.
INTERVIEWER: It's a chore? Right.
MISS HENDERSON: And you can get that feeling it is a chore, they're doing it because it's a job, they don't, not really doing it because they think they're helping you or whatever.
INTERVIEWER: Right, right.
MISS HENDERSON: You can, it is an attitude to work, I think.... I think, it is just a job to them. Way of earning money. Survival. Well, it comes to all of us doesn't it?
INTERVIEWER: Yes, well work's a bit like that, isn't it. So, when you say they're a bit brisk and brusque. Are they ever rough, or just with their words, or manner?
MISS HENDERSON: Well they're rough in their manner of speaking, some of them. And I'm sure it is because they've got a chip, chip on their shoulders.

It is important to recognise that racism is a complex phenomenon that does not operate in a unitary or wholly consistent way. People express contradictory and ambivalent views that often intersect with ideas of class (Law 1996). Feelings about black staff in the study were often mixed up with the problem of agency staff. In London it was difficult for social services to recruit workers and they were forced to use agencies where turnover tended to be high, and many of the workers only worked in the sector on a reluctant and temporary basis. These tensions were then negotiated through the categories of 'race'.

A number of clients went out of their way to be positive about black workers, and this was not simply as a prelude to later critical comments. Thus Mr Kirkwood remembering an excellent careworker said:

MR KIRKWOOD: We had a black man, was wonderful – ohh! [said to express delight].
MR BOYD: Yes, he was every so good, brilliant. We are not anti-black by any means.

Others, however, clearly felt that they had to be careful in making critical comments about black workers to social services in case their views were interpreted as racist. There was a general feeling that negative comments about individual black workers or about their attitudes would be poorly received by agencies or social services. This perception was broadly correct. In interviews with managers, 'race' was acknowledged to be an issue in London, but was treated exclusively as a problem of individual elderly white clients who were racist. No broader context of racial conflict or struggle was admitted, though these clearly mediated some of the exchanges between clients and workers, as the cases of Mrs Elster and Mrs Ostrovski show.

Mrs Elster was confined to her bed and in order for her to remain living at home in difficult circumstances, her routines were necessarily exacting. This created friction with careworkers who resented close direction and tried to evade her control, using techniques like hiding in the kitchen, forgetting her instructions, mumbling and refusing to hear when she called. Relations were therefore conflictual, marked by struggles around power and control. In Mrs Elster's view 'race' was an element in this. She commented: 'They are coloured, they won't do this and they won't do that'. Mrs Elster went on to emphasise that she was not 'anti-coloured' as such :

I've had two coloured girls who were marvellous ... and it's not with me a matter of colour ... it's the attitude ... I've got two Indian friends I've had for nearly 30 years, I knew them as students when they came from Calcutta, so it's not that I'm anti-colour, I'm anti-attitude yes, that very much so.

In this context of tension, certain actions that might otherwise have been neutral in character, took on a special and charged meaning, as the incident of the carpet illustrates. Mrs Elster was incontinent and from time to time the carpet at the front of her bed on which she sat and lay needed cleaning. In order to do this effectively, workers needed to kneel at her feet and give it a scrub. The resonances of this, however, were such that workers either refused to do the task or went about it in ways designed to minimise the denigrating character of the symbolism. As Mrs Elster explained:

> The other thing I've noticed with the coloured ladies is they won't kneel. Now this mat here because I'm incontinent some-times gets a drip or two, so once a week it has to be scrubbed ... None of them will get down on their hands and knees and do it, they sort of either stoop, or that way, or they squat and they get very cross ... Not a particularly good job but then other people never make any fuss about it, Trudy [a favoured white care-worker training to be a doctor] never blinked her eye and that kind of thing, just got on with it, on her hands and knees.

Race relations in Britain are embedded in a colonial past, and indeed a number of the clients in the London sample had lived part of their lives under colonial conditions: Miss Henderson was brought up in India, Mrs Fitzgerald had lived in Hong Kong, Sir Peter had served much of his career abroad. Careworkers were aware of this and at times of stress or conflict the existence of such a history added a charge to the relationship. Mrs Ostrovski who was Polish, resented such assumptions. Like Mrs Elster and Miss Henderson, she felt that Afro-Caribbean workers had a chip on their shoulder and resented her asking them to do things or correcting them. Mrs Ostrovski had a fairly pre-emptory manner in dealing with staff – something that I observed directly – that would have been resented across the board, but in the conditions of inter-racial relations this assumed a charged meaning. The matter may not have started with being about 'race', but it soon became so, and disputes escalated into references to slavery and other historical wrongs. Mrs Ostrovski recounted an incident when the careworker had failed to do something exactly as she had asked and when she pointed this out, replied, 'Don't talk to me like that. Don't think that I am your slave. Slavery has finished long ago.' Mrs Ostrovski reported how she replied:

> Well you are barking in the wrong tree. First of all I am not English and my grandfather didn't have any cotton plantation. I am from Poland and the one black man I saw, he was a porter in

a big hotel, so I have not seen – I did not see a black in my life, so don't tell me about my grandparents having a plantation and you being a slave.

In denying the relevance of that racial history of exploitation and servitude, however, she still managed to touch on a different, class-based set of tensions in which she was positioned as the hotel guest and the black worker as a servant.

Careworkers bring to the work their experiences of living and working in a racist society. On a day-to-day basis they are aware of the racialised nature of the labour market in which they work. Black people are differentially to be found in the least advantaged areas of employment, particularly low-level manual work in the public sector. Institutions like hospitals display a very clear racial hierarchy (Ward 1993). As we noted earlier these are workers who to some degree find that their choices are constrained. The history of black employment has in part been one of fitting into the jobs that other, more privileged and white workers, have rejected.

There are parallels here with the situation in the US where race is an even more significant factor and where the literature on carework reflects an altogether harsher employment world. In North America the home care workforce is differentially drawn from people of colour and immigrant groups (Donovan 1989, Feldman *et al* 1990, Neysmith and Aronson 1996). Black women in the US have historically been confined to the least desirable female jobs, concentrated in private household work and technologically backward sectors, and home care is part of this. Feldman and her colleagues found that race was a significant negative factor in job satisfaction, and they attribute this to both the racial harassment that black workers experience and the fact that a proportion of black workers find themselves confined, by reason of discrimination, lack of skills and educational opportunities, to work for which they are ill suited (Feldman *et al* 1990). Tellis-Nayak and Tellis-Nayak (1989) note the concern that is sometimes expressed in the US about a cold and unresponsive manner among many nursing home aides, but they argue that this needs to be set in the context of the social worlds from which these workers come, worlds where life is a daily struggle, where personal relations are sometimes violent and abusive, where the day-to-day realities of racism erode human responsiveness and where harsh attitudes and values are necessary for survival. If nursing home aides seem by middle class standards to be 'dispassionate and indifferent', it is because they have learnt life's lessons well.

The need to develop a tough, even harsh, personality, is described in accounts of the training of white residential careworkers in Britain too; Skeggs (1997) and Bates (1993) both regard schooling in the tougher versions of the working-class family as a necessary background for the job, so that this harshness is not about 'race' itself, but it can be mediated by the experience of 'race' and of living in a racist society. Some at least of the more transgressive group interviews appeared to contain such a feeling, where the group – made up of black workers – asserted themselves against the organisation but also, more significantly, against the white clients. In these interviews a rougher tone, and harsher attitude emerged, with disparaging remarks made about clients and about their bodies. We have already seen in Chapter 7 how workers used these as a means of getting their own back on clients for the work that they have to do. Black workers know that they are involved in doing menial work for white people, and that knowledge forms part of the background to their responses.

If we turn to the accounts given by the black and ethnic minority careworkers, most agreed that clients could be racist; and the majority had experienced racism in their day-to-day work. As Desiree recounted:

> I've been called a black monster [laughing] I've been told I'm gonna put her in the cooking pot and eat her. Doors have been shut in my face … it's not been actually said, but you know it's because you're black, they don't want you in.

This reflects the findings of the NISW study of the social services workforce where 40 per cent of the black and ethnic minority workers had experienced racist abuse from users relatively frequently or from time to time (Williams 1995). In the interviews most of the black careworkers rationalised such response in terms of the age of the clients and the worlds from which they had come. Their frailty was also constituted as something of an excuse. Most workers said that they shrugged off racist remarks. Zara who was one of Mrs Elster's workers recounted one incident:

> I went to a client's house and he needed a bath … and his wife opened the door for me and she went to him and she said to him like um, 'oh it's a girl, a woman' and he goes 'why do they keep always sending women', you know like he didn't want a woman. And then he goes 'what colour is she?' and I heard him, but she

was like, she must have said 'oh, she's black'. And he went like, 'why do they always send black people' … Most of the clients I've had, they're just easy going really. Whether you're black or white, you know. Long can do the job that's all that really matters to them. But then you do get the odd one and two that will be all, that probably voice their opinion, but it's never been directly to me, it's always been like, indirect, you know.

In general, black respondents agreed that it was best to ignore racist remarks, unless they were particularly flagrant. Zara:

If it's indirect it doesn't really bother me. I just shrug that off. Unless I hear, if I hear it and I find it offensive, then I'll be like 'oh, you're so cheeky, how can you say that', you know. But, I wouldn't let it bother me, I won't let it bother me really.

Neysmith and Aronson (1997) similarly found that careworkers downplayed the impact of racist remarks and tried not to allow themselves to be hurt by them. In the struggle for self esteem, dwelling on this sort of negativity is painful and personally draining.

For some black careworkers, their response to questions of 'race' was embedded in an implicit critique of white society, in which the dynamics were reversed and Britain constructed as the negative Other. Joshua, who came originally from Sierra Leone, perceived Britain as a country where old people were left to be cared for by strangers: 'In Africa … We don't have social care …. The relatives take care of their old people.' Britain was a place where terrible things like rape and paedophilia happened: 'In this country … some men are sick you know, like they rape old women 90 years old or 5 years old girl.' As a result, he felt, old people were fearful of strangers and agencies had to careful about staff. For him, and for some of the other black careworkers, caring was also located in the context of a religious response to life; and acting in a caring way was for him part of the stream of blessings in his life. Desiree, despite her fairly tough attitude to clients, also referred to religion in her account of her work: 'I believe that's what I was put here for – that's my mission from God to [do this work].'

Class

The relations of care are also mediated by class. Most of the classic accounts of home care rest on the situation where working-class women care for working-class clients, and this has underwritten the warm family-like relations that such studies typically describe (Warren 1988). But in many cases, the class relations of care are of a different, more discordant character. The study contained people from a variety of occupational backgrounds: a hospital porter, a Lyons nippy, a senior naval officer, the wife of a surgeon, the female director of a national charity, the widow of a builder, a gardener, a male clairvoyant, people who had been servants, as well as those who had had servants. Relations with the careworkers were thus mediated through a variety of class positions, though the impact of these was sometimes softened by the low incomes of many older people. Some of the respondents who had had upper-middle-class backgrounds and careers, and retained some of the mien of such, now lived in straitened circumstances.

How does class affect the power dynamics of care? First, it is clear that the family model of the relationship that many studies describe is largely inappropriate where there are considerable class differences. Very few clients in the study regarded the careworker as a daughter or other sort of relative; and those that did so, were more likely to share the same class background. (They were also more likely to be frail, emotionally dependent on the careworker and wanting to draw on the reserves of commitment that familial models suggest.) In the case of Mr Hedges who did describe Joshua as a son, this common class background was reinforced by 'race'. In most cases, careworkers were described either in terms of a professional doing a job, or a friend, or more correctly, as one respondent said, as 'friendly-like'. Similar processes worked in reverse. Working-class careworkers caring for upper-middle-class clients did not describe them in terms of being like their mothers or other relatives. Though relations sometimes took on something of the unbounded character of family obligation, as the struggles around 'extras' showed, this was a result of the dynamics of dependence rather than the power of the familial model. It was because people needed them that they did these things and got close to them, not because they constructed the relationship in terms of family.

Second, class affects the power that clients are able to bring to the exchange. Upper-middle-class respondents, as a result of their cultural capital in the sense used by Bourdieu, had greater resources to deploy in the dynamics of the care encounter. At the simplest level, they were accustomed to being helped; and earlier experiences with servants and other domestic assistance endowed them with a certain ease and social assurance in relation to domestic care. This class dimension was more marked among women than men. The traditional relations of gender in the family mean that men of all classes are accustomed to being supported and assisted in their day-to-day lives. It was among the women, especially working and lower-middle class women, that the experience of being helped was a new and often awkward one. To some degree this history of class confidence in relation to domestic help extended into the new experience of being helped in the bath. The pattern of embarrassment or unease around such intimate care was a complex and personal one, but there was a sense that the situation was easier for the upper-middle-class respondents. I do not think that this necessarily reflected a general attitude to the body as Featherstone and Hepworth (1991) argue, so much as a greater interpersonal confidence around being helped. As we saw in Chapter 3, Miss Garfield displayed some of this 'don't give a damn' feeling in her responses. When asked if a regular worker was nicer, she agreed that it made conversation easier but:

MISS GARFIELD: Really only from that point of view.... From the bathing point of view, I don't give a damn....
INTERVIEWER: Were you always someone who was kind of quite free and easy about these sorts of things, do you think? I mean some people are more modest than others I think, some people find it all rather ...
MISS GARFIELD: I'm afraid I'm not modest at all, you know. Why a grown person should be modest I don't know.

When asked if she got ready in any special way before the bath attendant came, she replied:

MISS GARFIELD: No I don't take any notice, poor things they have to put up with how it is. (Laughing)
INTERVIEWER: Right, so you're not having to kind of tidy up the bathroom and make it all nice?
MISS GARFIELD: Oh no, no, no. No nonsense like that.

All this was said in a confident take-it-or-leave-it tone.

Class differences mean that for some clients, the careworkers offered little in the way of companionship. This was important because many older people, who are housebound, are as much bored as lonely. Sir Peter was blind as well as physically frail, but his mind was active and he looked forward to any intelligent conversation that he could get. Mrs Elster found her current caregivers not very interesting to talk to, and she contrasted this with an earlier Swedish caregiver who had been training to become a doctor.

> I certainly am not a blue stocking but I'm just a little bit above them ... some of the words I use, they sort of look at me and say, 'What's that?' and so there's no way ... whatever you say to them however nice or nasty you are, they just say yes or no, grunt more than likely. So with again, Trudie, I could talk to her, we used to chat, when we were working mind you, we didn't just sit and chatter all the time.

How did the careworkers respond to these dynamics of class? The question of being treated like a servant was, as we have seen, a sensitive one, and rooted in class-based history of work identities. Zara clearly felt that class affected the attitudes of clients to her and to her work. For her there were two classes of people. Rich ones were more used to domestic labour, and insisted on their money's worth.

> I find with the rich people, when I was doing the home-help I found with them they want their money's worth.... So I have, I have realised that in the two different classes of wealth. The ones that don't have the wealth are the more easier going than the ones with the wealth.

They took a more commodified view of her labour, seeing it as something that had been allocated to and purchased by them, and open therefore to their direction.

Wealth and class differences also affected the degree to which workers felt at ease in the space of the home, as well as the warmth of the relationship. Bernadette, an Irish woman in her late forties, commented: 'It's always the people with money, I find the coldest'. She preferred caring for someone who was more her own class: she felt they treated her with greater respect and did not try to maintain social distance.

BERNADETTE: Any rich ones I've had, treat you with disrespect.
INTERVIEWER: Disrespect?
BERNADETTE: Yeah, I prefer poor, well not poor. People like meself, just living for the day. They've more respect for ya and they understand you more. They're more homely, you know what I mean.

She clearly preferred a relationship that was more socially equal and where the client did not keep a distance. This is an important aspect in the power dynamics of care. As we have seen, careworkers resent clients who maintain their autonomy and refuse to give them emotional access, and this is more likely to happen where relations of class underwrite distance, thus denying workers some of their emotional rewards.

For Barry, the structures of class and gender intersected. Status was an important issue for him. Though he valued and enjoyed carework, he was conscious of the poor esteem in which it was held, particularly for a man. This came out in his relations with male clients, some of whom had been powerful figures in the public world, and who he felt despised him for doing this work, denying him the status as an equal. There was a gender as well as class element in this, reflecting the competitive nature of men's relations with other men.

> I think it's far harder working with somebody who used to be extremely wealthy or extremely powerful. We get all sorts. We get sort of former politicians and all that sort of thing. Sort of high up military men. And it's extremely difficult because they've always had everything done for them, they've got this great expectation, and they don't see you so much as – *they don't see you as an equal at all.* And that's far harder to take. The hardest thing about being a carer sometimes isn't the emotional sort of difficulties within the job, it's the stigma and the view that other people have of you.

In dealing with these powerful and wealthy men, it was difficult to get them to see him as an equal, or to get to know them on a closer basis: 'it is definitely harder and there are some people you can't get that close to.' Withholding closeness was once again an element in the dynamics of power. Barry was very conscious how such denial of closeness and equality was linked to being treated like a servant, something that he felt was demeaning:

> Because no one ever sees themselves as being a slave or as being underneath somebody else. I mean, you are an individual in your own right, and everyone's equal. There's some people you go in to and you're not. You just have to sell your soul for ninety minutes when you're in their house.

As we have noted these dynamics of personal service apply most strongly to cleaning work. Once the work involves body care, however, the relationship inevitably changes, for before the needs of the body, as Barry explained, even the grandest person is humbled:

> The actual sort of personal care or bathing, it does actually sort of transcend that. I used to go in and see some sort of extremely wealthy people. I used to sort of see a former politician every day, twice a day. And it would still be that, [ie social superiority and distance] underneath the surface, absolutely no doubt about it. But you could certainly – it would certainly be more sort of equal. It would be sort of a partnership, but I imagine if I was going in there for something else, it would be extremely sort of master, servant, relationship. Because if you're putting your faith in somebody's hands, if you're sort of hoisting somebody out of bed twice a day, or sort of making sure they can do the most basic things ... Humbling is perhaps the wrong word, but it does sort of get rid of any sort of difference between two people.

Doing intimate personal care allows the worker to break through the client's barrier of superiority, and assert their equality with the grandest.

> You know, on the commode [pauses] you can't see people and say, well you can't physically treat them in that sort of distant off-handish way, you know, for a client. It's get rid of any baggage.... It probably does belittle the person really. It probably gets rid of their power.

Bodycare does ultimately reduce people, even the previously powerful, and workers know this.

Conclusion

Bathing is a site of conflict, where both workers and clients struggle for self esteem and control. Workers extract forms of payment from clients over and above those represented in the job agreement. Clients are expected to show gratitude, and to give back to workers some of the emotional rewards that they seek in the work; and failing to do so is a breach of the implicit care contact. Distant clients who maintain their independence, and resist intimacy, or who attempt to assert a relationship of control, are disliked and sometimes made subject to punishment in the form of the withdrawal of attention. Treating the careworker like a servant, or the home like a hotel, is a breach of the implicit emotional contract. Clients are expected to be 'needy' and the reward for this is care, including care that sometimes goes beyond the formal requirements of the job. Attempts to claim this care by right, however, on a consumerist model are resented; as are attempts to push the boundary beyond the discretionary point fixed by the worker. This is seen as taking advantage, and resisted.

Workers sometimes refuse to do tasks that they dislike even though they are officially part of the job. In London, careworkers sometimes avoid heavy cleaning which they regard as onerous and beneath them and they exert power over clients to shape the work in ways that they like. This does not always happen, and cleaning work does get done, but it is not the straightforward expectation that it might seem to be from the outside. It has to be negotiated. Cleaning work is in general disliked, and careworkers prefer to downplay these aspects of their work, emphasising care instead. Carework is preferred because it has greater status, being nearer the professional model of nursing, and because it allows the worker to establish dominance. This dominance may not always be exercised directly, and it can have an indirect nurturant quality to it, but it is dominance all the same. The intimacy of bodywork is significant here. It is hard for clients to maintain psychological autonomy and distance where the contact is so direct and personal. The worker is right there next to them, handling their body and directing their movements. Bodywork is transgressive and involves forms of exposure that can be embarrassing and that reduces individuals in their own and others' eyes. It is particularly hard to assert independence in the face of things like incontinence; and levels of expressed gratitude rise in line with the embarrassment or humiliation of the interventions.

Clients struggle unequally with these forces of domination. The power that they can exert in the exchange is limited. Largely they are forced to rely on the good will of the workers, underpinned by the organisational framework that defines the official nature of the job. Those who are wise may themselves engage in emotional labour in reverse, implicitly recognising the parallel system of 'payment' that exists in the form of gratitude, warmth and acknowledged dependence. Careworkers are often individuals who value neediness in others and derive a sense of esteem from being able to respond to it. The price of accepting this can however be high, and infantalisation is rife in carework.

These issues of power and dominance are mediated through structures of class and race. White upper-middle-class clients are able to bring to the care encounter cultural capital acquired over their earlier lives. Sometimes this capital takes the material form of the surroundings in which they live – the power of home as a crystallisation of identity – but often it is in the form of a social manner or habit of confidence, something that itself helps create the desired response. This manner can however be resented, and careworkers resist strongly any attempts by the client to assert a master/servant style relationship. Rejecting the status of a servant is at the heart of the power struggle of care, and it is the direct personal subordination implied by such a role that is resisted and denied. It is for this reason that models of good practice that attempt to assert a version of care in which the client is wholly in charge rarely succeed. Community care cannot be wholly separated from the historical roots that give such activities their definition.

Carework is similarly mediated through structures of 'race'. Clients believe that 'race' is a significant factor. Sometimes they express this directly though the medium of racist discourse in relation to the body. Other times it is less direct and intersects with other features of the London labour market, in particular its transient character. Clients will sometimes describe such workers as rough, uncaring and with a chip on their shoulder. 'Race' in Britain is embedded in a colonial past, and this brings added resonance to its power dynamics. Questions of dominance, of master and servant, are refracted through the lens of this history and assume an additional and more charged set of meanings as a result. As a result, kneeling or not kneeling to scrub the carpet comes to have a larger significance.

Conclusion

There are three main themes in this book. The first concerns the experience and management of the body, and how this is refracted through the lenses of race, class, age and gender. Bodywork takes place in the silenced areas of western culture and this contributes to its experience from both sides. The second addresses the ambivalences of the body, how these are managed in the care encounter, and how they are carried over into the uncertain forms of closeness that are created by care. The third is the significance of the day-to-day and mundane in people's lives, and the centrality of this for the study of community care and more widely.

We have seen how the body lies at the heart of community care, both from the perspective of older and disabled people and careworkers. Community care *is* bodycare. The experiences of the body and care are mediated through structures of age, gender, race and class. Careworkers and clients bring to the care encounter sets of experiences and cultural assumptions that derive from the wider social world, and these profoundly affect the nature of the exchange. Among these experiences are those of 'race'. We saw in the last chapter how carework can become entangled with issues of 'race', and how the struggle for control and self-esteem on both sides can be given an additional twist by virtue of the existence of histories of colonial domination. Furthermore black and ethnic minority careworkers find themselves systemically located in disadvantaged sectors of the labour market, where the rewards are poor and the status low. They are more likely to be employed in the rougher, more coercive, parts of the care system, and they bring to their working lives the day-to-day experience of living in a racist society. Past histories are thus played out in current practice.

These structures of 'race' intersect with those of class; and many of the tensions that arise in relation to 'race' find their counterpart in class. Most work on home care has assumed a shared culture between working-class women workers and their clients of similar background. But this is not always the case. Clients do not always share the same social world as workers, and this can put constraints on the warmth and interest of the relationship. Through the use of class distance, clients can also treat careworkers in such a way as to deny them emotional access, and with that some of the key rewards of carework. Gratitude and emotional openness are part of the implicit care contract, and failure to show them undermines the nature of the relationship as conceptualised by the careworkers – a relationship in which clients are needy and careworkers caring. Class can also enable clients to activate elements of the servant model that careworkers are at pains to resist – keeping emotional distance, directing their work, deploying the confidence that derives from a lifetime of class advantage. Their capacity to do this is however severely limited, and their frailty means that workers in general have the upper hand. Personal care is indeed a great watershed in status. To move across that boundary, to be helped in these areas, is to lose a great deal of one's social power, and few individuals manage to maintain their authority in these circumstances. Care is fundamentally an unequal power relationship.

Gender similarly profoundly affects the nature of the care encounter. We saw how the bodies of men and women are treated differently in culture, and how this supports different expectations and conventions around the provision of care, particularly in regard to cross-gender tending. As so often in relation to the body – and indeed gender more generally – this operates in an asymmetrical way; and the meaning for men of receiving care from a woman (or a man) is different from that of a woman receiving help from a man (or a woman). This reflects the wider gendered treatment of the body and sexuality in culture, in which women's bodies are constructed in terms of male desire, and modesty and decorum are imposed and internalised as part of the wider control of sexuality. This has consequences for the differential way in which women experience their bodies, both when they are younger, and in the context of disability and old age. Gender is also central in the construction of carework. This is a job that – like nursing – is formed around the attributes of femininity; and this underpins its character as both bodywork and emotional labour. Many of the conflicts that characterise carework come from its gendered character, in particular the tensions that arise when care as an activity that has been socially defined within the structures of home and the private sphere is transferred into the public sphere of employment and economic rationality. In other words, when the unbounded ethic of care meets and clashes with the formal demands of waged labour.

That care is about age is so obvious as to be often overlooked. It is commonplace for books exploring the social structure of society to discuss the intersecting dimensions of Class, Race and Gender, but Age is only rarely included. This is despite the fact that is the most profoundly influential of them all. We live our whole lives on a journey through age. At every stage its structures determine our experiences. It is so profoundly part of existence, that we often neglect to mention it. Society is stratified in terms of age; and age structures are among the most significant in determining the meanings of what we do and the likely receptions we will meet. Age is particularly central in the experience of the body. Though chronological age does not predict bodily state, the two are linked. Receiving help with personal care marks one of the great watersheds of the aging process, one of the profound changes that marks the Ages of Man, or Woman. As we saw, most elderly respondents in the study accepted such changes in a stoical way, seeing raging against them as unproductive and painful. For the workers too, age is a significant subject; and carework brings them directly up against the realities of their own futures, requiring them to ponder the mystery of aging: the fact that as the clients are now, so too will they one day be. For some this was a disturbing thought that they sought to push away. For others the exercise in imagination was too great. Though they knew intellectually that the old bodies that they now cared for had once been young, they found it hard to grasp on an emotional level.

We have seen how the body in old age and disability contains a number of ambivalences, and how these centre around the 'negativities of the body' – incontinence, decay, bodily failure generally. Managing such aspects is awkward and embarrassing from both sides, and their presence gives a particular character to the encounter. Personal care is transgressive, both in that it deals with such negativities, and that it disturbs the normal pattern of social intimacy. Personal care involves nakedness and touch, forms of closeness that go beyond what is customary for non-erotic relationships; and this creates, as we saw, a strange form of intimacy, one in which closeness is necessary and to some degree valued, but at the same time is a source of unease. There was a discordant element in this closeness; and, by and large, the physical intimacy of personal care is not welcomed as a route to greater emotional closeness.

Workers sometimes attempt to put boundaries on the extent of this closeness; and this applies both to the physical aspects of carework and the emotional ones. Care with its unbounded ethic of love and its powerful undertow of emotional connectedness, contains the potential to engulf the worker. Setting limits on this is a necessary part of surviving the job.

These ambivalences apply to the recipients also. Personal care creates a strange and disjunctive form of intimacy. By and large, people prefer that it take place within a defined and specific relationship, not one that had a prior existence, such as a friend or relation. In the eyes of those people, clients prefer to remain the person they always were, and that by and large means someone with their clothes on, managing their own bodily functions. Personal care breaches the normal social order, and people prefer to compartmentalise its provision if they can. For some, however, this is not possible, and care increasingly dominates and takes over their lives, so that the structures of care come to be the structures of daily life.

Lastly this book contains a plea for the role of the ordinary and the mundane in the analysis of community care and more widely. It is in the day-to-day structures of people's lives, with their rhythms and regularities, that much of the meaning lies. Bathing and washing are part of this, and we saw how such practices have historically encapsulated a range of social symbolism and significance. Day-to-day existence, including bodily existence, is at the heart of our lives. This is true for all of us, but is perhaps most true for people as they approach their latter years, when the structures of work no longer make a claim, and when – for some at least – life has become more closely condensed around the home. Social and public policy needs to get a grip on these dimensions if its prescriptions are to have any purchase on the day-to-day realities of care.

Appendix
The study

The study was based on qualitative interviews with older and disabled people and with careworkers and front line managers that aimed to explore the experiences of receiving and giving help with bathing and washing. The research was undertaken in two areas: a relatively wealthy part of inner London and a deprived coastal area. The class structure of the sample reflected these differences, with the London group including a number of upper-middle-class people, as well as those from other backgrounds. The Coastville group were more mixed, and included a majority from lower-middle and working-class backgrounds. Thirty recipients of bathing help were included in the study, though in three cases, owing to dementia, their carers responded on their behalf. Interviews were undertaken with carers and family members where appropriate. In four cases, these interviews were joint. The majority of the sample were older people, though five younger physically disabled people were also interviewed. Twenty-one recipients were female and nine male. The sample was recruited via voluntary sector agencies and social services. All names are anonymised.

The interviews with careworkers and other staff were undertaken in a mixture of one-to-one and group interviews. Thirty-four careworkers were interviewed: thirty-one were female and three male. They were employed by a variety of agencies: social services, private for profit and voluntary sector. Four community nurses (one male), three day centre staff, and five front-line managers were interviewed.

I am grateful to Economic and Social Research Council of the UK for funding the study under grant R000236731.

References

Abbott, P. (1994) 'Conflict over the grey areas: district nurses and home helps providing community care', *Journal of Gender Studies*, 3, 3, 299–306.

Acker, J. (1990) 'Hierarchies, jobs and bodies: a theory of gendered organisations', *Gender and Society*, 4, 2, 139–58.

Adam, B. (1995) *Timewatch: the Social Analysis of Time*, Cambridge: Polity.

Adkins, L. (1995) *Gendered Work: Sexuality, Family and the Labour Market*, Buckingham: Open University Press.

Ahmad, W.I.U. and Atkin, K. (eds) (1996) *'Race' and Community Care*, Buckingham: Open University Press.

Allan, G. (1989) 'Insiders and outsiders: boundaries around the home', in G. Allan and G. Crow (eds) *Home and Family: Creating the Domestic Sphere*, London: Macmillan.

Allan, G. and Crow, G. (eds) (1989) 'Introduction', in G. Allan and G. Crow (eds) *Home and Family: Creating the Domestic Sphere*. London: Macmillan.

Andrews, M. (1999) 'The seductiveness of agelessness', *Ageing and Society*, 19, 301–18.

Ardener, S. (1987) 'A note on gender iconography: the vagina', in P.Caplan (ed.) *The Cultural Construction of Sexuality*, London: Routledge.

Aronson, J. and Neysmith, S.M. (1996) ' " You're not just there to do the work": depersonalizing policies and the exploitation of home care workers' labor', *Gender and Society*, 10, 1, 59–77.

Baker Miller, J. (1978) *Towards a New Psychology of Women*, Harmondsworth: Penguin.

Balbo, L.(1987) 'Crazy quilts: rethinking the welfare state debate from a woman's point of view', in A. Showstack Sassoon (ed.) *Women and the State: the Shifting Boundaries of Public and Private*, London: Hutchinson.

Baldock, J. (1997) 'Social care in old age: more than a funding problem', *Social Policy and Administration*, 31, 1, 71–89.

Baldock, J.(1998) 'Old age, consumerism and the social care market', in E. Brunsdon, H. Dean and R. Woods (eds) *Social Policy Review 10*, London: SPA.

Baldwin, S. (1997) 'Charging users for community care', in M. May, E. Brunsdon, G. Craig (eds) *Social Policy Review 9*, London: SPA.

Balloch, S., McLean, J. and Fisher, M.(eds) (1999) *Social Services: Working Under Pressure*, Bristol: Policy Press.

Bartoldus, E., Gillery, B. and Stuges, P. J. (1989) 'Stress and coping among home-care workers', *Health and Social Work*, 14, August, 204–10.

Bashford, A. (2000) *Purity and Pollution: Gender Embodiment and Victorian Medicine*, Basingstoke: Macmillan.

Bates, I. (1993) 'A job which is "right for me"?: social class, gender and individualisation', in I. Bates and G. Riseborough (eds) *Youth and Inequality*, Buckingham: Open University Press.

Bauman, Z. (1992) *Intimations of Postmodernity*, London: Routledge.

Beardsworth, A. and Keil, T. (1997) *Sociology on the Menu: An Invitation to the Study of Food and Society*, London: Routledge.

Belk, R.W. (1992) 'Attachment to possessions', in I. Altman and S.M. Low, (eds) *Place Attachment*, New York: Plenum Press.

Bell, D. and Valentine, G. (1997) *Consuming Geographies: We Are What We Eat*, London: Routledge.

Bendelow, G. and Williams, S.J. (eds) (1998) *Emotions in Social Life: Critical Themes and Contemporary Issues,* London: Routledge.

Benjamin, A.E. (1993) 'An historical perspective on home care policy', *Milbank Quarterly*, 71, 1, 129–66.

Berger, P. L.(1973) *The Social Reality of Religion*, Harmondsworth: Penguin.

Bergson, H. (1910) *Time and Free Will: An Essay on the Immediate Data of Consciousness*, London: Macmillan, trs F.L.Pogson.

Bird, P. (1995) 'The origins of Victorian public baths, with special reference to Dulwich baths', *The Local Historian*, August, 142–52.

Bordo, S. (1993) *Unbearable Weight: Feminism, Western Culture and the Body*, Berkeley: University of California Press.

Brown, H. and Smith, H. (eds) (1992) *Normalisation: A Reader for the Nineties*, London: Routledge.

Burbridge, L.C. (1993) 'The labor market for home care workers: demand, supply and institutional barriers', *The Gerontologist*, 33, 1, 41–6.

Burnett, J. (1974) *Useful Toil: Autobiographies of Working People from the 1820s–1920s*, London: Allen Lane.

Bury, M. (1995) 'The body in question', *Medical Sociology News*, 21, 1, 36–48.

Bushman, R. L. and Bushman, C. L.(1988) 'The early history of cleanliness in America', *Journal of American History*, 74, 4, 1213–38.

Business and Research Associates (1986) 'The UK market for bathroom equipment', BRA: London.

Butler, J. P. (1993) *Bodies that Matter: On the Discursive Limits of 'Sex'*, London: Routledge.

Chapman, T. and Lucas, R. J. (1998)' "A place to live": portrayals of body privacy and communion in contemporary show homes', paper given at 1998 BSA conference, Making Sense of the Body, Edinburgh.

Clark, H., Dyer, S. and Horwood, J. (1998) *'That bit of help': The High Value of Low Level Preventative Services for Older People,* Bristol: Policy Press.

Clark, K. (1956) *The Nude: A Study of Ideal Art*, London: John Murray.

Clark, S. (1994) *Japan: a View from the Bath*, Honolulu: University of Hawaii Press.

Charles, N. and Kerr, M. (1988) *Women, Food and Families*, Manchester: Manchester University Press.

Classen, C., Howes, D. and Synnott, A. (1994) *Aroma: The Cultural History of Smell*, London: Routledge.

Connell, R.W. (1995) *Masculinities*, Cambridge: Polity.

Corbin, A. (1986) *The Foul and the Fragrant: Odor and the French Social Imagination*, Leamington Spa: Berg.

Daatland, S. (1990) 'What are families for?: On family solidarity and preference for help', *Ageing and Society*, 10, 1–15.

Daunton, M. J. (1983) *House and the Home in the Victorian City: Working Class Housing 1850–1914*, London: Edward Arnold.

Davies, B. and Challis, D. (1986) *Matching Resources to Needs in Community Care: An Evaluated Demonstration of a Long Term Care Model*, Aldershot: Gower.

Davies, C. (1995) *Gender and the Professional Predicament in Nursing*, Buckingham: Open University Press.

—— (1998) 'Caregiving, carework and professional care' in A. Brechin, J. Walmsley, J. Katz and S. Peace (eds) *Care Matters: Concepts, Practice and Research in Health and Social Care*, London: Sage.

Davies, K. (1994) 'The tensions between process time and clock time in carework: the example of day nurseries', *Time and Society*, 3, 3, 277–303.

Davis, K. (1995) *Reshaping the Female Body: The Dilemma of Cosmetic Surgery*, London: Routledge.

—— (ed.) (1997) *Embodied Practices: Feminist Perspectives on the Body*, London: Sage.

Dexter, M. and Harbert, W. (1983) *The Home Help Service*, London: Tavistock.

Diamond, T. (1988) 'Social policy and everyday life in nursing homes: a critical ethnography', in A. Statham, E.M. Miller and H.O. Manksch (eds) *The Worth of Women's Work*, Albany, NY: SUNY.

—— (1992) *Making Gray Gold: Narratives of Nursing Home Care*, Chicago: University of Chicago Press.

Dominelli, L. (1992) 'An uncaring profession? An examination of racism in social work', in P. Braham, A. Rattansi and R. Skellington (eds) *Racism and Antiracism: Inequalities, Opportunities and Policies*, London: Sage.

Donovan, R. (1989) ' "We care for the most important people in your life": Home care workers in New York city', *Women's Studies Quarterly*, 1&2, 56–65.

Douglas, M. (1966) *Purity and Danger: An Analysis of the Concepts of Pollution and Taboo*. London: Routledge and Kegan Paul.

—— (1970) *Natural Symbols*, Harmondsworth: Penguin.

—— (1975) 'Jokes', in *Implicit Meanings: Essays in Anthropology*, London: Routledge and Kegan Paul.

Dunlop, M (1986) 'Is a science of caring possible?' *Journal of Advanced Nursing,* 11, 661–70.

Elias, N. (1978) *The Civilizing Process: The History of Manners,* Oxford: Blackwell.

Ellis, K and Dean, H. (eds) (2000) *Social Policy and the Body: Transitions in Corporeal Discourses,* Basingstoke: Macmillan.

Emerson, R.M. and Pollner, M. (1976) 'Dirty work designations: their features and consequences in a psychiatric setting', *Social Problems,* 23, 243–54.

Estes, Carroll L. and Binney, Elizabeth A.(1989) 'The biomedicalization of aging', *The Gerontologist,* 29, 5, 587–96.

Eustis, N.N., Fischer, L.R. and Kane, R.A. (1994) 'The home care worker: on the front line of quality', *Generations,* XVIII, 3, Fall.

Eustis, N.N., Kane, R.A. and Fischer, L.R. (1993) 'Home care quality and the home care worker: beyond quality assurance as usual', *The Gerontologist,* 33, 1, 64–73.

Featherstone, M. (1991) 'The body in consumer culture', in M. Featherstone, M. Hepworth and B.S. Turner (eds) *The Body: Social Process and Cultural Theory,* London: Sage.

Featherstone, M. and Hepworth, M. (1991) 'The mask of ageing and the postmodern life course', in M. Featherstone, M. Hepworth and B.S. Turner (eds) *The Body: Social Process and Cultural Theory,* London: Sage.

Featherstone, M. and Wernick, A. (eds) (1995) *Images of Aging: Cultural Representations of Later Life,* London: Routledge.

Feldman, P. H. (1993) 'Work life improvements for home care workers: impact and feasibility', *The Gerontologist,* 33, 1, 47–54.

Feldman, P.H., Sapienza, A.M. and Kane, N.M. (1990) *Who Cares for Them: Workers in the Home Care Industry,* New York: Greenwood Press.

Ferlie, E., Challis, D. and Davies, B. (1989) *Efficiency-Improving Innovations in Social Care of the Elderly,* Aldershot: Gower.

Ferlie, E., Ashburner, L., Fitzgerald, L. and Pettigrew, A. (1996) *The New Public Management in Action,* Oxford: Oxford University Press.

Finch, J. (1989) *Family Obligations and Social Change,* Cambridge: Polity.

Finch, J. and Groves, D. (eds.) (1983) *A Labour of Love: Women, Work and Caring,* London: Routledge.

Finch, J. and Mason, J. (1993) *Negotiating Family Responsibilities,* London: Routledge.

Fineman, S. (1993) 'Organisations as emotional arenas', in Fineman, S. (ed.) (1993) *Emotion in Organisation,* London: Sage.

Firth, R. (1973) *Symbols: Public and Private,* London: Allen and Unwin.

Fitzgerald, M. and Sim, J. (1979) *British Prisons,* Oxford: Blackwell.

Floyer, Sir John (1706) *The History of Cold Bathing: Both Ancient and Modern,* London.

Ford, J., Quilgars, D. and Rugg, J. (1998) *Creating Jobs: the Employment Potential of Domiciliary Care,* Bristol: Policy Press.

Foucault, M. (1973) *The Birth of the Clinic: An Archaeology of Medical Perception,* London: Tavistock.

—— (1977) *Discipline and Punish: The Birth of the Prison*, Harmondsworth: Allen Lane.

—— (1979) *The History of Sexuality, Volume I*, Harmondsworth: Penguin.

Furman, F. K. (1997) *Facing the Mirror: Older Women and Beauty Shop Culture*, New York: Routledge.

Game, A. (1995) 'Time, space and memory, with reference to Bachelard', in M. Featherstone, S. Lash and R. Robertson (eds) *Global Modernities*, London: Sage.

Gennep, A. van (1908) *The Rites of Passage*, translated by M.B.Vizedom and G.L. Cafee (1960), London: Routledge and Kegan Paul.

Gershuny, J. (1978) *After Industrial Society: The Emerging Self-Service Economy*, Basingstoke: Macmillan.

Giddens, A. (1991) *Modernity and Self-Identity: Self and Society in the Late Modern Age*, Cambridge: Polity.

Giedion, S. (1948) *Mechanization Takes Command*, New York: Oxford University Press.

Gilligan, C. (1982) *In a Different Voice: Psychological Theory and Women's Development*, Cambridge: Harvard University Press.

Gimlin, D. (1996) 'Pamela's place: power and negotiation in the hair salon', *Gender and Society*, 10, 5, 505–26.

Ginn, J. and Arber, S. (1993) 'Ageing and cultural stereotypes of older women' in J. Johnson and R. Slater (eds) *Ageing and Later Life*, London: Sage.

Girouard, M. (1979) *The Victorian Country House*, London: Yale.

Glendinning, C., Schunk, M. and McLaughlin, E. (1997) 'Paying for long-term domiciliary care: a comparative perspective', *Ageing and Society*, 17, 123–40.

Goffman, E. (1961) *Asylums: Essays on the Social Situations of Mental Patients and Other Inmates*, New York: Doubleday.

—— (1969) *The Presentation of Self in Everyday Life*, Harmondsworth: Penguin.

Goubert, J.-P. (1989) *The Conquest of Water: the Advent of Health in the Industrial Age*, Cambridge: Polity.

Graham, H. (1991) 'The concept of caring in feminist research: the case of domestic service', *Sociology*, 25, 1, 61–78.

Greer, G. (1986) *The Madwoman's Underclothes: Essays and Occasional Writings 1968–85*, London: Picador.

Gregson, N. and Lowe, M. (1994) *Serving the Middle Classes: Class, Gender and Waged Domestic Labour in Contemporary Britain*, London: Routledge.

Gubrium, J.F. (1975) *Living and Dying in Murray Manor*, New York: St Martins.

Gurney, C.M. (1998) 'Accommodating bodies: theorising the body in housing studies', paper given at 1998 BSA conference, Making Sense of the Body, Edinburgh.

Gurney, C.M. and Means, R. (1993) 'The meaning of home in later life', in S. Arber and M. Evandriou (eds) *Ageing, Independence and the Life Course*, London: Jessica Kingsley.

Hantrais, L. (1993) 'The gender of time in professional occupations', *Time and Society*, 2, 2, 139–57.

Harvey, D. (1989) *The Condition of Postmodernity*, Oxford: Blackwell.

Health and Safety Executive (1992) *Manual Handling: Guidance on Regulations*, London: HMSO.

Hembry, P. (1990) *The English Spa, 1560–1815: A Social History*, London: Athlone Press.

—— (1997) *British Spas from 1815 to the Present: A Social History*, London: Athlone Press.

Henley, N.M. (1973) 'The politics of touch', in P. Brown (ed.) *Radical Psychology*, London: Tavistock.

Higgins, J. (1989) 'Homes and institutions', in G. Allan and G. Crow (eds) *Home and Family: Creating the Domestic Sphere*, London: Macmillan.

Hochschild, A. (1983) *The Managed Heart: The Commercialisation of Human Feelings*, Berkeley, CA: University of California.

Hochschild, A. (1993) 'Preface', in S. Fineman (ed.) *Emotion in Organisation*, London: Sage.

Hughes, B. and Paterson, K. (1997) 'The social model of disability and the disappearing body: towards a sociology of impairment', *Disability and Society*, 12, 3, 325–40.

Huntingdon, J. (1981) *Social Work and General Medical Practice*, London: Allen and Unwin.

Illich, I. (1976) *Limits to Medicine, Medical Nemesis, the Expropriation of Health*, London: Boyars.

Isaacs, B. and Neville, Y. (1976) 'The needs of old people: the "interval" as a method of measurement', *British Journal of Preventative and Social Medicine*, 30, 79–85.

James, N. (1989) 'Emotional labour: skill and work in the social regulation of feelings', *Sociological Review*, 1, 15–42.

James, N. (1992) 'Care organisation and physical labour and emotional labour', *Sociology of Health and Illness*, 14, 4, 488–509.

James, V. and Gabe, J. (eds) (1996) *Health and the Sociology of Emotions*, Oxford: Blackwell.

Jordanova, L. (1989) *Sexual Visions: Images of Gender in Science and Medicine between the Eighteenth and Twentieth Centuries*, Hemel Hempstead: Harvester Wheatsheaf.

Jourard, S.M. (1966) 'An exploratory study of body accessibility', *British Journal of Social and Clinical Psychology*, 5, 221–31.

Jourard, S.M. and Rubin, J.E. (1968) 'Self disclosure and touching: a study of two modes of interpersonal encounter and their inter-relation', *Journal of Humanistic Psychology*, 8, 1, 39–48.

Katz, S. (1996) *Disciplining Old Age: the Formation of Gerontological Knowledge*, Charlottesville: University Press of Virginia.

Kestenbaum, A. (1996) *Independent Living: A Review*, York: Joseph Rowntree Foundation.

Kilito, A. (1993) 'Architecture and the sacred: a season in the hammam', *Research in African Literatures*, 23, 2, 203–08.

Kira, A. (1967) *The Bathroom: Criteria for Design*, New York: Bantam.

Kontos, P.C. (1999) 'Local biology: bodies of difference in ageing studies', *Ageing and Society*, 19, 6, 677–89.

Koren, L. (1996) *Undesigning the Bath*, Berkeley, CA: Stone Bridge Press.

Laing, H. and Laing A. (nd) 'History', in M. Binney (ed.) *Taking the Plunge: The Architecture of Bathing*, London: Save Britain's Heritage.

Laing, W. and Saper, P. (1999) 'Promoting the development of a flourishing independent sector alongside good quality public services', in *With Respect to Old Age, Research Volume 3*, Cm 4192-II/3, London: The Stationery Office.

Larabee, M.J. (ed.)(1993) *An Ethic of Care: Feminist and Interdisciplinary Perspectives*, London: Routledge.

Largey, G.P. and Watson, D.R (1972) 'The sociology of odors', *American Journal of Sociology*, 77, 6, 1021–33.

Law, I. (1996) *Racism, Ethnicity and Social Policy*, London: Prentice Hall.

Lawler, J. (1991) *Behind the Screens: Nursing, Somology and the Problem of the Body*, Melbourne: Churchill Livingstone.

Lawler, J. (1997) 'Knowing the body and embodiment: methodologies, discourses and nursing.', in J. Lawler (ed.) *The Body in Nursing*, Melbourne: Churchill Livingstone.

Lawrence, C. (1998) 'Medical minds and surgical bodies: corporeality and the doctors,' in C. Lawrence and S. Shapin (eds) *Science Incarnate: Historical Embodiments of Natural Knowledge*, Chicago: University of Chicago Press.

Lawrence, R.J. (1987) *Housing, Dwellings and Homes: Design Theory, Research and Practice*, Chichester: Wiley.

Lawton, J. (1998) 'Contemporary hospice care: the sequestration of the unbounded body and "dirty dying" ', *Sociology of Health and Illness*, 20, 2, 121–43.

Leccardi, C. (1996) 'Rethinking social time: feminist perspectives', *Time and Society*, 5, 2,169–86.

Leccardi, C. and Rampazi, M. (1993) 'Past and future in young women's experience of time', *Time and Society*, 2, 353–80.

Lee-Treweek, G. (1994) 'Bedroom abuse: the hidden work in a nursing home', *Generations Review*, 4, 1, 2–4.

—— (1996) 'Emotion work, order and emotional power in care assistant work', in V. James and J. Gabe (eds) *Health and the Sociology of the Emotions*, Oxford: Blackwell.

—— (1998) 'Women, resistance and care: an ethnographic study of nursing auxiliary work,' *Work, Employment and Society*, 11, 1, 47–63.

Lévi, P. (1987) *If This Is a Man*, London: Abacus.

Lévi-Strauss, C. (1970) *The Raw and the Cooked: Introduction to a Science of Mythology Volume I*, London: Cape.

—— (1973) *From Honey to Ashes: Introduction to a Science of Mythology Volume II*, London: Cape.

—— (1978) *The Origin of Table Manners: Introduction to a Science of Mythology Volume III*, London: Cape.

Lewis, G. (2000) 'Introduction: expanding the social policy imaginary', in G. Lewis, S. Gewirtz and J. Clarke (eds) *Rethinking Social Policy*, London: Sage.

Lewis, J. and Meredith, B. (1988*) Daughters who Care: Daughters Caring for Mothers at Home,* London: Routledge.

Lewis, J. and Glennerster, H. (1996) *Implementing the New Community Care*, Buckingham: Open University.

Littlewood, J. (1991) 'Care and ambiguity: towards a concept of nursing', in P. Holden and J. Littlewood (eds) *Anthropology and Nursing*, London: Routledge.

Lonsdale, S. (1990) *Women and Disability: The Experience of Physical Disability Among Women*, Basingstoke: Macmillan.

Lovenduski, J. and Randall, V. (1993) *Contemporary Feminist Politics: Women and Power in Britain*, Oxford: Oxford University Press.

Lupton, D. (1994) *Medicine as Culture: Illness, Disease and the Body in Western Societies,* London: Sage.

—— (1996) *Food, the Body and the Self,* London: Sage.

McCorkle, R. and Hollenbach, M. (1984) 'Touch and the actutely ill' in C.C. Brown (ed.) *The Many Facets of Touch*, New Brunswick: Johnson and Johnson.

MacSween, M. (1993) *Anorexic Bodies: A Feminist and Sociological Perspective on Anorexia Nervosa*, London: Routledge.

Martin, E. (1987) *The Woman in the Body*, Milton Keynes: Open University.

Mason, J. (1989) 'Reconstructing the public and the private: the home and marriage in later life', in G. Allan and G. Crow (eds) *Home and Family: Creating the Domestic Space*, London: Macmillan.

Maugham, W.S. (1922) *On a Chinese Screen*, London: Heinemann.

Mauss, M. (1973, 1934) 'Techniques of the body', *Economy and Society,* 2, 70–88.

Means, R. and Smith, R. (1985) *The Development of Welfare Services for Elderly People*, London: Croom Helm.

Merquior, J.G. (1985) *Foucault*, London: Fontana.

Miller, W. I. (1997) *The Anatomy of Disgust*, Cambridge, Mass.: Harvard University Press.

Minkler, M. and Estes, C.L. (eds) (1991) *Critical Perspectives on Aging, the Political and Moral Economy of Growing Old*, Amityville, NY: Baywood.

Montagu, A. (1986) *Touching: the Human Signifiance of Skin*, 3rd ed., New York: Harper & Row.

Morgan, D (1993) 'You too can have a body like mine: reflections on the male body and masculinities', in S.Scott and D. Morgan (eds) *Body Matters: Essays on the Sociology of the Body*, London: Falmer Press.

Morris, J. (1993) *Independent Lives: Community Care and Disabled People*, Basingstoke: Macmillan.

—— (1997) 'Care or empowerment? A disability rights perspective', *Social Policy and Administration*, 31, 1, 54–60.

Mulkay, M. (1988) *On Humour: Its Nature and Its Place in Modern Society*, Cambridge: Polity.

Munro, M. and Madigan, R. (1993) 'Privacy in the private sphere', *Housing Studies*, 8, 1, 29–45.

Murcott, A. (1982) 'On the Social Significance of the "cooked dinner" in South Wales', *Social Science Information*, Vol. 21, 677–96.

—— (ed.) (1983) *The Sociology of Food and Eating*, Aldershot: Gower.

Nettleton, S. and Watson, J. (eds) (1998) *The Body in Everyday Life*, London: Routledge.

Neysmith, S. M. and Aronson, J (1996) 'Home care workers discuss their work: the skills required to "use your common sense" ', *Journal of Aging Studies*, 10,1, 1–14.

Neysmith, S. M. and Aronson, J. (1997) 'Working conditions in home care: negotiating race and class boundaries in gendered work', *International Journal of Health Services*, 27, 3, 479–99.

Nirascou, G. (1998) 'Propreté: les clignotants sont au gris', *Le Figaro*, 20 Novembre, 12.

Obelkevich, J. (1994) 'Consumption', in J. Obelkevich and P. Catterall (eds) *Understanding Post-war British Society*, London: Routledge.

Öberg, P. (1996) 'The absent body – a social gerontological paradox', *Ageing and Society*, 16, 6, 701–19.

Oliver, M. (1990) *The Politics of Disablement*, Basingstoke: Macmillan.

Orwell, G. (1937, 1962) *The Road to Wigan Pier*, Harmondsworth: Penguin.

Parker, G. (1993) *With This Body: Caring and Disability in Marriage*, Buckingham: Open University.

Parker, G. and Seymour, J. (1998) 'Male carers in marriage: re-examining feminist analyses of informal care', in J. Popay, J. Hearn and J. Edwards (eds) *Men, Gender Divisions and Welfare*, London: Routledge.

Pearson, M.P. and Richards, C. (1994) 'Ordering the world: perceptions of architecture, space and time', in M.P. Pearson and C. Richards (eds) *Architecture and Order: Approaches to Social Space*, London: Routledge.

Phillipson, C. and Walker, A. (eds) (1986) *Ageing and Social Policy: A Critical Assessment*, Aldershot: Gower.

Porter, S. (1992) 'Women in a woman's job: the gendered experience of nurses', *Sociology of Health and Illness*, 14, 4, 510–27 .

Pringle, R. (1989) *Secretaries Talk: Sexuality, Power and Work*, London: Verso.

PSSRU (1998) *Bulletin: Evaluating Community Care for Elderly People*, Canterbury: Kent.

Rabinow, P. (ed.) (1984) *The Foucault Reader: An Introduction to Foucault's Thought,* Harmondsworth: Penguin.

Raverat, G. (1952) *Period Piece: A Cambridge Childhood*, London: Faber & Faber.

Reverby, S.M. (1987) *Ordered to Care: the Dilemma of American Nursing, 1850–1945*, Cambridge: Cambridge University Press.

Riet, P. van der (1997) 'The body, the person, technologies and nursing', in J. Lawler (ed.) *The Body in Nursing*, Melbourne: Churchill Livingstone.

Ritzer, G. (1993) *The McDonaldization of Society*, Thousand Oaks: Pine Forge Press.

Ross, K. (1995) *Fast Cars, Clean Bodies: Decolonialization and the Reordering of French Culture*, Cambridge, Mass.: MIT Press.

Rostgaard, T. and Fridberg, T. (1998) *Caring for Children and Older People: A Comparison of European Policies and Practices. Social Security in Europe 6*, Copenhagen: Danish National Institute of Social Research.

Rousseau, J.J. (1764) *Emile, or On Education*, trans. A. Bloom (1978) Harmondsworth: Penguin.

Routasalo, P. and Isola, A. (1996) 'The right to be touch and be touched', *Nursing Ethics*, 3, 2, 165–76.

Royal Commission on Long Term Care (1999) 'Lessons from international experience'. In *With Respect to Old Age – Rights and Responsibilities: The Context of Long Term Care Policy: Research Volume I*, Cm 4192-II/1, London: The Stationery Office.

Rubinstein, R.L. (1989) 'The home environments of older people: a description of the psychosocial processes linking person to place', *Journal of Gerontology*, 44, 2, S45–53.

Rubinstein, R.L. and Parmelee, P.A. (1992) 'Attachment to place and the representation of the life course by the elderly', in I. Altman and S.M.Low (eds) *Place Attachment*, New York: Plenum Press.

Savage, J. (1995) *Nursing Intimacy: An Ethnographic Approach to Nurse–Patient Interaction*, London: Scutari Press.

Scull, A. (1993) *The Most Solitary of Afflictions: Madness and Society in Britain 1700–1900*, London: Yale.

Shakespeare, T. (1994) 'Cultural representations of disabled people: dustbins for disavowal', *Disability and Society*, 9, 3, 283–99.

Sharma, U. and Black, P. (1999) 'The sociology of pampering: beauty therapy as a form of work', Derby: University of Derby, Centre for Social Research Working Paper.

Sheridan, A. (1980) *Michel Foucault: The Will to Truth*, London: Routledge.

Shilling, C. (1993) *The Body and Social Theory*, London: Sage.

Sinclair, I., Parker, R., Leat, D. and Williams, J. (1990) *The Kaleidoscope of Care: A Review of Research on Welfare Provision for Elderly People*, London: HMSO.

Sixsmith, A. (1990) 'The meaning and experience of "home" in later life', in B. Bytheway and J. Johnson (eds) *Welfare and the Ageing Experience*, Aldershot: Avebury.

Skeggs, B. (1997) *Formations of Class and Gender: Becoming Respectable*, London: Sage.

Smart, C. (1989) *Feminism and the Power of Law*, London: Routledge.

Smith, H. and Brown, H. (1992) 'Inside-out: a psychodynamic approach to normalisation', in H. Brown and H. Smith (eds) *Normalisation: A Reader for the Nineties*, London: Routledge.

Social Services Inspectorate (1987) *From home help to home care, an analysis of policy, resources and service Management*, London: Department of Health and Social Security.

Sussman, N.M. and Rosenfeld, H.M. (1978) 'Touch, justification and sex: influences on the aversiveness of spatial violations', *Journal of Social Psychology*, 106, 214–25.

Swenarton, M. (1977) 'Having a bath: English domestic bathrooms, 1890–1940', in *Leisure in the Twentieth Century: History of Design*, London: Design Council Publications.

Synnott, A (1993) *The Body Social: Symbolism, Self and Society*, London: Routledge.

Tellis-Nayak, V. and Tellis-Nayak, M. (1989) 'Quality of care and the burden of two cultures: when the world of the nursing aide enters the world of the nursing home', *Gerontologist*, 29, 3, 307–13.

Tester, S. (1996) *Community Care for Older People: A Comparative Perspective*, Basingstoke: Macmillan.

Thackeray, W.M. (1848) *The History of Pendennis*, London: Bradbury & Evans.

Thomas, C. (1993) 'De-constructing concepts of care', *Sociology*, 27, 4, 649–69.

Thompson, E.P. (1967) 'Time, work discipline and industrial capitalism,' *Past and Present*, 36, 52–97.

Tomes, N. (1998) *The Gospel of Germs: Men, Women and the Microbe in American Life*, Cambridge, Mass.: Harvard University Press.

Townsend, P. (1986), 'Ageism and social policy', in C. Phillipson and A. Walker *Ageing and Social Policy: A Critical Assessment*, Aldershot: Gower.

Townsend, P. and Davidson, N. (eds) (1982) *Inequalities in Health: The Black Report*, Harmondsworth: Penguin.

Tronto, J.C. (1993) *Moral Boundaries: A Political Argument for an Ethic of Care*, London: Routledge.

Turner, B.S. (1984) *The Body and Society: Explorations in Social Theory*, Oxford: Blackwell.

—— (1991) 'Recent developments in the theory of the body', in M. Featherstone, M. Hepworth and B.S. Turner (eds) *The Body: Social Process and Cultural Theory*, London: Sage.

—— (1997) 'From govermentality to risk: some reflections on Foucault's contribution to medical sociology', in A. Petersen and R. Brunton (eds) *Foucault: Health and Medicine*, London: Routledge.

Turner, V.W. (1969) *The Ritual Process: Structure and Anti-structure*, Harmondsworth: Penguin.

Twigg, J. (1983) 'Vegetarianism and the meaning of meat', in A. Murcott (ed.) *The Sociology of Food and Eating: Essays in the Sociological Significance of Food*, Aldershot: Gower.

—— (1997) 'Deconstructing the "social bath": help with bathing at home for older and disabled people', *Journal of Social Policy*, 26, 2, 211–32.

—— (2000) 'Social policy and the body', in G. Lewis, S. Gewirtz and J. Clarke (eds) *Rethinking Social Policy*, London: Sage.

Twigg, J. and Atkin, K. (1994) *Carers Perceived: Policy and Practice in Informal Care*, Buckingham: Open University.

Ungerson, C. (1983) 'Women and caring: skills, tasks and taboos', in E. Gamarnikow, D. Morgan, J. Purvis and D. Taylorson (eds) *The Public and the Private*, London: Heinemann.

—— (1987) *Policy Is Personal: Sex, Gender and Informal Care*, London: Tavistock.

—— (ed.) (1990) *Gender and Caring: Work and Welfare in Britain and Scandinavia*, London: Wheatsheaf.

—— (1993) 'Payment for caring: mapping a territory', in N. Deakin and R. Page (eds) *The Costs of Welfare*, Aldershot: Avebury.

—— (1999) 'Hybrid forms of work and care: the case of personal assistants and disabled people', *Work, Employment and Society*, 13, 4, 583–600.

Urry, J. (1996) 'Sociology of time and space', in B.S. Turner (ed.) *The Blackwell Companion to Social Theory*, Oxford: Blackwell.

Vigarello, G. (1988) *Concepts of Cleanliness: Changing Attitudes in France Since the Middle Ages*, Cambridge: Cambridge University Press.

Waerness, K. (1987) 'On the rationality of caring', in A. Showstack Sassoon (ed.) *Women and the State: the Shifting Boundaries of Public and Private*, London: Hutchinson.

Walby, S. (1990) *Theorizing Patriarchy*, Oxford: Blackwell.

Walker, A. and Warren, L. (1996) *Changing Services for Older People*, Buckingham: Open University Press.

Wall, A. (ed.) (1996) *Health Care Systems in Liberal Democracies*, London: Routledge.

Ward, L. (1993) 'Race, equality and employment in the NHS', in W.I.U. Ahmad (ed.) *Race and Health in Contemporary Britain*, Buckingham: Open University.

Ward, L. and Philpot, T. (eds) (1995) *Values and Visions: Changing Ideas in Services for People with Learning Difficulties*, Oxford: Butterworth-Heinemann.

Warde, A. (1997) *Consumption, Food and Taste*, London: Sage.

Warren, L. (1988) 'Home care and elderly people: the experience of home helps and older people in Salford', PhD thesis presented at the University of Salford.

—— (1994) 'Tradition and transition: the role of the support worker in community care in Sheffield', in D. Challis, B. Davies and K. Traske (eds) *Community Care: New Agendas and Challenges from the UK and Overseas*, London: Arena.

Watson, J. (2000) *Male Bodies: Health, Culture and Identity*, Buckingham: Open University Press.

Wharton, A.S. (1993) 'The affective consequences of service work: managing emotions on the job', *Work and Occupations*, 20, 2, 205–32.

Whitcher, J.S. and Fisher, J.D. (1979) 'Multidimensional reaction to therapeutic touch in a hospital setting', *Journal of Personality and Social Psychology*, 37, 1, 87–96.

Wiles, R. (1993) 'Women and private medicine', *Sociology of Health and Illness*, 15, 1, 68–85.

Wilkie, J.S. (1986) 'Submerged sensuality: technology and perceptions of bathing', *Journal of Social History*, summer, 649–54.

Wilkin, D. and Hughes B. (1987) 'Residential care of elderly people: the consumer's views', *Ageing and Society*, 7, 2, 175–202.

Williams, C.L. (1989) *Gender Differences at Work: Women and Men in Non Traditional Occupations*, Berkeley: University of California Press.

Williams, J. (1995) 'Black staff in social services', in S. Balloch, T. Andrew, J. Ginn, J. McLean, J. Pahl and J. Williams (eds) *Working in Social Services*, London: National Institute for Social Work.

Williams, M.T. (1991) *Washing the 'Great Unwashed': Public Baths in Urban America, 1840–1920*, Columbus, Ohio: Ohio State University Press.

Williams, S.J. and Bendelow, G. (1998) *The Lived Body: Sociological Themes, Embodied Issues*, London: Routledge.

Wistow, G., Knapp, M., Hardy, B. and Allen, C. (1994) *Social Care in a Mixed Economy*, Buckingham: Open University Press.

Wistow, G., Hardy, B., Young, R., Forder, J., Kendall, J. and Knapp, M. (1997) 'Purchasing home care: how independent sector providers see the developing market', *Evidence: Briefing Paper Two*, Leeds: Nuffield Institute for Health.

Wolf, N. (1990) *The Beauty Myth: How Images of Beauty Are Used Against Women*, London: Vintage.

Wolf, Z.R. (1988) *Nurses' Work, the Sacred and Profane*, Philadelphia: University of Pennsylvania Press.

Wolkowitz, C. (1998) 'Conceptualising the body in body work occupations and contexts', paper given at Work, Employment and Society Conference, Cambridge.

Wood, Roy C. (1995) *The Sociology of the Meal*, Edinburgh: Edinburgh University Press.

Wright, L. (1960) *Clean and Decent: the Fascinating History of the Bathroom*, London: Routledge.

Yegül, F. (1992) *Baths and Bathing in Classical Antiquity*, Harvard: MIT Press.

Young, I.M. (1990) *Throwing Like a Girl and Other Essays in Feminist Philosophy and Social Theory*, Bloomington: Indiana University Press.

Index

touch 47–8, 58–9, 61–3, 139,
  150–52
Tronto, J.C. 172
Turner, B.S. 8, 17, 39

Ungerson, C. 71–2, 156, 193
uniforms 124, 150, 192

Vigarello, G. 28

Waerness, K. 9, 97
Warren, L. 130, 191, 202
washing 25–8; *see also* bathing
Wharton, A.S. 162
Williams, C.L. 131
Wolkowitz, C. 140

Young, I.M. 9